Road transport and health

British Medical Association

September 1997

A publication from the BMA Science Department

Chairman, Board of Science and Education:	Professor Jack Howell
Head, Professional Resources and Research Group:	Professor Vivienne Nathanson
Editors:	Dr David R Morgan Sallie Robins
Consultant Writer:	Adrian Davis (Health and Transport Research Group, School of Health and Social Welfare, Open University)
Editorial Secretariat:	Lisa Davies Hilary Glanville Hayley Todd
Indexer:	Richard Jones
Design:	Hilary Glanville

British Library Cataloguing in Publication Data
A catalogue record for this book is available from the British Library

ISBN 0 7279 1197 X

First published in 1997 by: British Medical Association, Tavistock Square, London, WC1H 9JP

Printed by: The Chameleon Press, London

Acknowledgement

Thanks are due to the following copyright owners for permission to reproduce their photographs: Andrew Tryner, Rural Development Commission, Michael Hancock, Rural Development Commission, BMA News Review, The Transport Research Laboratory, Lisa Davies.

Contents

1 Introduction

British Medical Association and Board of Science and Education

The British Medical Association (BMA) is a professional organisation representing all doctors in the UK. It was established in 1832 to *promote the medical and allied sciences, and to maintain the honour and interests of the medical profession.* The BMA Board of Science and Education supports this aim by providing an interface between the profession, the government, and the public, and by undertaking research studies on behalf of the BMA. Through the publication of policy statements, the Board of Science and Education has led the debate on key public health and professional issues.

The overriding objective of the Board of Science and Education is to contribute to the development of better public health policies that affect the community, the state, and the medical profession. In order to do this, investigations are carried out by the Board to examine the impact of various policies and activities on the public health. The Board appoints working parties and steering groups, combining medical and other specialist expertise, to carry out research on a variety of important issues. The Board has published a large number of reports over recent years reflecting current concerns in the public health arena such as pesticides, transport policy, complementary medicine and environmental and occupational hazards of the health service.

The Board also has responsibility for educational initiatives. Many of the reports published through the Board are used in medical not only develops such educational materials but also has an interest in educational policy, and most recently examined the education of doctors in multicultural health care.

Transport policy and the BMA

At the BMA's 1995 Annual Representative Meeting (ARM) it was resolved: *that this meeting calls upon the BMA to define and develop a clear policy for transport and its likely impact on health and the environment.* As the Board of Science and Education had already established a working party to examine the environmental impact of certain projects including those related to transport, it was decided in relation to this resolution, that the Board should focus on the health impact of transport. It was also decided to focus on road transport as this part of the transport sector potentially had the greatest impact on health. Although the BMA has undertaken much work in relation to transport and health, this has primarily focused on accident prevention or reduction and the BMA has established policy in relation to drinking and driving, seat belt legislation, and cycling.

Transport as a health issue

The primary function of transport is the movement of people and goods between places, enabling access to people, social activities and leisure, goods and services. Ease of access is essential for both the nation's economy and human health and wellbeing. How access needs are met determines whether the health of individuals and the public is promoted or damaged.

In general, the influences on health of transport policy that receive the greatest attention are those of road traffic accidents and increasingly, air pollution. These more quantifiable influences are of great importance, but there are a broad range of other factors that need to be considered.

The wide range of positive and negative influences that transport may have on health are summarised below:

Enabling access to:	Traffic injuries
employment	Pollution:
shops	carbon monoxide
recreation	nitrogen oxides
social support networks	hydrocarbons
health services	ozone
countryside	lead
Recreation	benzene
Physical activity	particulate matter
	Noise and vibration
	Stress and anxiety
	Danger
	Loss of land and planning blight
	Severance of communities by roads

Source: Public Health Alliance. *Health on the Move: Policies for health promoting transport — Policy statement of the Transport and Health Study Group.* Birmingham: PHA, 1991

Depending on mode of travel used, transport can make a positive contribution to the national strategy for health, entitled *The Health of the Nation* (1992). *The Health of the Nation*[1] established for the first time a clear strategy for health in England and Wales, identified five key areas for action and set national objectives for these. These key areas were:

- Coronary heart disease and stroke

- Cancers

- Mental illness

- HIV/AIDS and sexual health

- Accidents

Transport can have benefits for at least three of the five *Health of the Nation* key areas, by reducing coronary heart disease and strokes, mental illness, and accidents and there is evidence for a reduction in cancer of the colon also. These benefits are largely associated with increased levels of aerobic physical activity which can be achieved through walking and cycling. In addition, a reduction in reliance on motorized forms of transport may improve mental health and wellbeing from less traffic noise, less driving stress, and improved local social support networks.

It is difficult to establish quantitative data for the health effects of transport policy such as the severance of communities or the benefits to mental health. This report therefore discusses the issues in general terms in order to highlight the number of ways in which transport may directly or indirectly affect both individual and public health. A broad range of recommendations are made which emphasise the need for an integrated transport policy and these have four key aims:

- reducing reliance on, and need for, health damaging forms of transport,

- increasing the use of health promoting forms of transport,

- increasing mobility and access and reducing inequity,

- reducing the negative effects of modes of transport.

Doctors and other health professionals have an important role in advocating healthy transport choices. They range from an individual general practitioner's (GP's) advice on a more physically active lifestyle, involving walking or cycling, to the broader role of public health doctors in addressing the health impact of transport policy in their locality. Collectively, the medical profession can have much influence in terms of promoting healthy public policy in relation to transport.

This report aims to promote broader debate of transport policy and health and highlight to the profession, public and government the many adverse effects that certain policies may have. Despite a key focus on the adverse effects of transport policy on health, there are a number of ways in which a new approach to transport policy may actually promote health. Developing strategies for preventing ill health, particularly at the population level is a key focus of the work of the BMA's Board of Science and Education and this document extends this work further into new policy areas.

were as follows:

Sir Donald Acheson	President, BMA
Dr S J Richards	Chairman of the Representative Body, BMA
Dr A W Macara	Chairman, BMA Council
Dr W J Appleyard	Treasurer, BMA
Professor J B L Howell	Chairman, Board of Science and Education
Dr P H Dangerfield	Deputy Chairman, Board of Science and Education
Dr J M Cundy	
Dr H W K Fell	
Miss C E Fozzard	
Dr E Harris	
Dr N D L Olsen	
Ms S Somjee	
Dr P Steadman	
Dr S Taylor	
Dr D Ward	

We are grateful for further expert guidance provided by
Dr W S Morton, Director of Public Health, East Lancashire Health
Authority, and Ms L Sloman, Assistant Director, Transport 2000.
We have been greatly assisted by the work the Transport and Health
Study Group has already done, in drawing together a body of
knowledge in this research area.

2 Patterns of transport use in Great Britain

Introduction

Within Great Britain, large increases in the number of journeys made and distances travelled have occurred over the past few decades. Modes of transport have also changed with rapidly increasing motorisation. In terms of kilometres travelled per head of population, the car (including taxis) is used more than any other mode of transport and Great Britain has the highest proportion of its passenger traffic travelling by car within the European Union countries.[2] Other modes have been in rapid decline, particularly cycling. In 1951 people in Great Britain cycled nearly 21 billion kilometres on public roads, which accounted for around a quarter of all road traffic. This fell rapidly to a low of 3.7 billion kilometres in 1973. In 1994 people cycled around 4.4 billion kilometres, only just over a fifth of the amount in 1951 and representing only 1% of all road traffic. Miles walked have also declined, on average, by 17% between 1975/76 and 1992/94 although 29% of all journeys are still made by foot. The number of journeys made by local bus has also declined, almost halving since 1971[3] (see Figure 1).

Mode of freight transportation has changed in the last four decades. Railways were the most important mode of transport for freight in 1952, but this has declined substantially and road transport of freight has increased four fold since 1952 (see Figure 2).[4] Heavy Goods Vehicles (HGV's) on roads now account for 80% of British freight, and rail transportation 7%.[5]

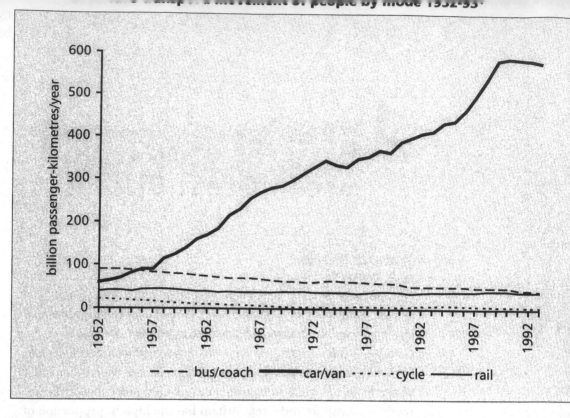

One noticeable change of transport use is the increase in car use for very short journeys that began in the late 1970s and 80s — increasing from 3.8% to 6.9% of all journeys of less than half a mile, and up from 14.7% to 24.1% of journeys between half a mile and a mile. As a proportion of all car journeys those of under a mile have increased from 6.4% of car journeys to 8.2%. It is likely that if account is taken of starting up, parking etc, the time by car for these journeys would not be all that different to the time taken to walk and almost certainly longer than the time taken to cycle.[6] Cycling is the quickest mode of transport in central and inner London.[7] In fact the majority of UK trips are relatively short — 72% of all trips being under five miles in length, however, 59% of such trips are made by car.[8] In terms of time spent travelling approximately 80% is spent travelling by car.

Social and entertainment journeys, such as visiting friends or taking part in sport make up the largest percentage of journeys (25%) with commuting, shopping and other personal business forming the

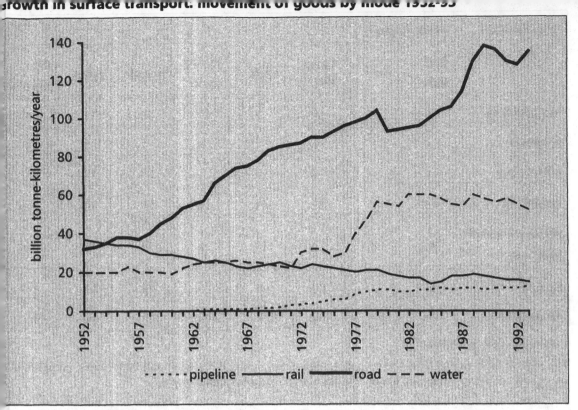

The coverage of statistics of waterborne freight was extended in 1972 and now includes north Sea oil traffic and other one-port freight movements.

second largest (19%). Commuting accounted for nearly 20% of the total distance travelled in Great Britain 1992-1994[3] (see Table 1).

Since the late 1980s the average number of journeys made on business has increased by a third, and these journeys now represent over a tenth of distance travelled.[9] This may be explained by the increase in the number of workers without a fixed place of employment. There have also been major changes in the way people shop. Between 1960 and 1981, one seventh of new retail floor space opened was at out of town sites, this rose to more than one half between 1982 and 1992.[10]

Increasing volumes of traffic are illustrated by data on flow of vehicles. Between 1981 and 1994 there was an increase of nearly 50% in the average daily flow of vehicles on roads in Great Britain and congestion on the roads is estimated to cost industry £19 billion per annum.[6]

Great Britain	Percentages							
	Car/ Van	Rail*	Local Bus	Walk	Motor- cycle	Bicycle	Other	All Modes
Commuting	18	49	20	9	48	38	11	19
Business	6	7	1	1	4	3	4	5
Education	2	7	14	10	1	10	19	5
Shopping	19	9	33	23	12	11	10	20
Other personal business	24	7	12	14	8	9	14	21
Leisure	31	21	20	44	27	29	41	31
All purposes	100	100	100	100	100	100	100	100

* Includes London Underground

NB: Figures refer to percentage of journey stages where a new stage is defined when there is a change of vehicle requiring a separate ticket. Figures exclude journeys under one mile.

Car use

Trends in car ownership are indicative of increasing motorization. Car ownership rose from 5.7 million in 1960 to about 23 million in 1995.[11] In some groups the increase has been particularly rapid. The percentage of women owning cars has increased nearly threefold between the years 1975-76 and 1992-94. In 1994-95 around 66% of households in Great Britain had a car or van available to them. In households headed by a professional over 50% have access to two or more cars.

Car use is now reported to be a necessity for many people rather than one of a range of modes of travel available, as it provides access, speed and convenience.[12] Many people are reliant on cars for certain necessary journeys where alternatives are simply not available at the time and place required. Even stronger constraints exist for some disabled people. Other factors leading to this

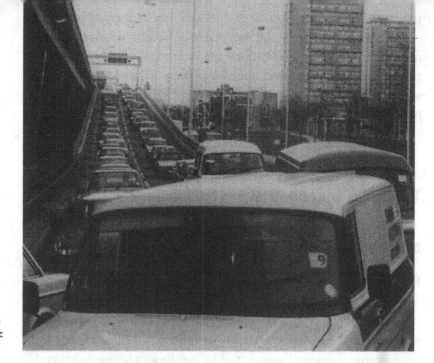

In Great Britain between 1981-1994 the average daily flow of road traffic increased by 50%.

dependence include the difficulties of managing travel with children, the need to carry heavy shopping, fears for safety on the streets and the lack of information about available alternatives.[6]

Heavy goods vehicles

Heavy goods vehicles (HGV) on roads now account for 80% of Britain's freight transport compared to only 7% on the rail system.[5] The 1989 National Road Traffic Forecasts predicted that HGV traffic could grow by 140% by 2025 under the high forecast figures.[4] Studies have shown that road freight has a much higher primary energy consumption of 2890 KJ/tonne-kilometre compared to 677 KJ/tonne-kilometre by rail, and the number of injuries per billion tonnes-kilometre has been estimated as 248 for road freight and 10 for rail freight.[4] However, at present the UK tax system favours road freight and makes it relatively cheap. Amounts paid in taxation by UK operators of HGV are substantially less than the costs their operators impose by way of environmental damage and requirements for infrastructure. The effect of this underpricing has been to distort competition in favour of road freight and encourage this, in 1974 the Department of Transport set up a grant scheme for companies to encourage the movement of freight to rail, to maximise the environmental benefits by removing lorries from roads. Regrettably however, take up of these grants has been low with just £32 million out of the budgeted £70 million being paid out between 1985 and 1995, this has been blamed on the demanding eligibility conditions and the time taken to process the applications.

Tackling increasing motorization

Demand vs supply

Road traffic is predicted to nearly double by 2025 (1988 baseline),[13] and despite the economically driven curtailments to the roads programme, traffic growth continues at roughly 3% per year. Even with the small expansion of network capacity that the 1989 roads programme envisaged, supply will be insufficient to meet demand. In addition, measures to reduce the adverse impacts of cars such as emission controls will be outweighed by the increasing number of motor vehicles. It is now widely accepted that it is neither environmentally acceptable nor economically possible to meet this demand for road space. Demand management and reducing the need to travel are now policy goals. Planning Policy Guidance Note 13 (PPG 13)[14] provides guidance to local authorities on the integration of transport and land-use planning. The key aims of PPG 13 are to reduce growth in the length and number of motorized journeys; encourage alternative means of travel which have less environmental impact; and hence reduce reliance on the private car.

Edinburgh City Council have recently unveiled their new 'Greenways' scheme which is intended to encourage a modal shift away from the car to public transport by decreasing local bus journey times. The first phase of the scheme involves painting the roads of two major routes within Edinburgh green and using single or red double lines to indicate that traffic cannot stop. Only buses, taxis and cyclists will be allowed to enter these green lanes during the designated hours. Buses will also be given traffic light setting priority. During the second phase, another three major routes within Edinburgh will be designated 'Greenways'. The cost for both phases is estimated at £15 million and a further £8 million has been invested in commissioning 68 low emission buses.

Support for alternatives

Current trends suggest that reliance on health damaging forms of transport is growing, and at a time when, for both individual and public health reasons, an increase in the use of health promoting forms of travel could ameliorate growing pressures in both the health and transport sectors. All the important trends reflect increasing volumes of motor traffic, especially in the countryside,[15] with the consequent environmental decline and increasing risk to individual and public health. Public opinion survey responses reflect this, perceiving environmental quality to be on the decline.[16,17] Research suggests that the public is supportive of more investment in alternatives to the car, and importantly that when given information about traffic growth, and cost effectiveness for various measures, support for restraint measures rises strongly, while support for increased spending on road/parking capacity declines.[18] In 1995 the British Social Attitudes survey asked people in Great Britain about their attitudes towards policy options for cars. The two most popular options for improvement amongst those surveyed were; reserving streets in towns and cities for pedestrians, and giving cyclists and pedestrians priority in towns and cities even if this makes things more difficult for other road users. Nearly 70% of individuals supported the former measure and just over 60% the latter.[19]

Over the past 5 decades, the pattern of road travel in Great Britain changed significantly. There has been a large increase in the number of journeys made and distances travelled and the modes of transport have also shifted away from walking, cycling and public transport, towards the motor car.

In 1951, cycling accounted for nearly 25% of all road traffic but by 1994 this figure had fallen to just 1%. Miles walked has also declined, on average, by 17% between 1975/76 and 1992/94. The car is now used more than any other mode of transport in Great Britain and between 1981 and 1984 there was an increase of nearly 50% in the average daily flow of motor vehicles on the roads. Cars are mainly used for social and entertainment journeys but more people now also rely on their car for commuting and for shopping at larger out of town complexes. The movement of freight by heavy goods vehicles (HGV) rather than rail, has also made a significant contribution to the increase in motor traffic.

It is predicted that the increase in road traffic will continue, although it is widely accepted that it is neither environmentally acceptable nor economically possible to meet the demand for road space. Research suggests that the public are supportive of measures to reduce traffic growth because environmental quality is perceived to be in decline. The emphasis in transport policy is therefore to reduce reliance on the motor car and to promote other forms of transport that are less environmentally damaging and may promote health.

3 The health benefits of road transport policy

Introduction

The fact that transport policy can influence health is increasingly recognised and the key mechanism by which people can benefit is through increasing their level of physical activity. Cycling and walking can be used as key means of transport, whether as a singular mode or as part of a journey incorporating other forms of transport because even use of public transport generally involves a certain amount of walking that door to door transport by car does not. For many reasons, levels of cycling and walking have been in decline in the UK. This chapter examines the potential for increasing levels of physical activity through walking and cycling and discusses the mechanisms for halting the decline in these important modes of transport.

Physical activity

There is a large body of research evidence relating physical activity to improvements in health status. The clear links between sedentary lifestyles and ill health were highlighted in the government strategy for health *The Health of the Nation*.[1] Lack of physical activity was identified as one of the four major risk factors for coronary heart disease and stroke. However, over seven in ten men and eight in ten women fall below their 'age appropriate activity' level necessary to achieve a health benefit.[20] There is therefore potential to reduce the high rates of coronary heart disease in the UK by increasing

and opportunities.[22] There is also evidence that the prevalence of obesity in Britain, which has doubled in the last decade, is as much due to the increasingly sedentary lifestyles of the population as to diet, and that inactive lifestyles may represent the dominant factor.[23] The Department of Health, as part of *The Health of the Nation* initiative, has developed a national physical activity strategy,[24] and transport is highlighted as a key policy area through which levels of physical activity could be raised.

Walking

Walking is the one mode of transport available to the majority of the population regardless of income, age, or location. It is non-polluting, consumes negligible natural resources, is highly efficient in its use of urban space and energy, and rarely causes injury to others and is still the most popular mode of travel after the car.

Figure 3
The decline in walking[25]

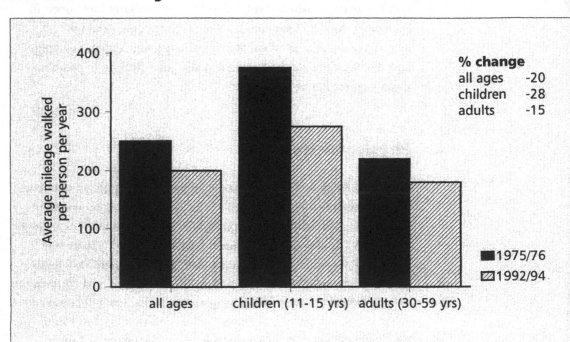

year has fallen from 239 in 1972/74 to 199 in 1992/94 — an overall decrease of 20%[8] (see Figure 3).

Health benefits of walking

There is now a consensus that regular moderate physical activity as part of the routine of daily living can provide the greatest public health benefit because vigorous activity is an unrealistic goal for the majority of the population. Statements by the Department of Health,[24] the World Health Organization/International Federation of Sports Medicine[26] and the Surgeon General in the United States[27] have highlighted the importance of regular moderate physical activity building up to at least five 30 minute bouts a week. Brisk walking, as a moderate intensity aerobic activity, provides the baseline level of protection required to confer significant health benefits.

Regular walking is important in cardiovascular disease prevention and management, and in the retention of function in late middle age and beyond. Of 9,000 civil servants between the ages of 45-64, the 9% of men who graded their walking as 'fast' experienced less than half the non-fatal and fatal coronary heart disease events than those who took no physical activity. Those assessing their walking to be 'fairly brisk' had less than two-thirds the rates for coronary attacks during the course of the nine year study.[28] Similar findings on the value of walking and the increased protection from disease as energy expended increases, have been reported elsewhere.[29] Research from Finland corroborates such findings, suggesting that journeys to and from work by foot meet the intensity criterion of physiologically effective physical activity for fitness and health.[30,31]

The ability to walk comfortably at a reasonable pace is important for independence and quality of life. Older people, especially post-menopausal women, have a specific need to continue regular, rhythmic, weightbearing exercise, to preserve bone mineral density against osteoporosis, protect against hypertension and stroke, and maintain the integrity of muscle function and physical confidence essential to the avoidance of falls and consequent hip fractures.[32] Regular moderate activities such as brisk walking improve strength, flexibility, speed of muscle contraction, muscle endurance, gait and

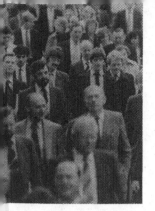

Walking, as part of the routine of daily living, can provide a significant health benefit.

importance for men as the protective effect of testicular hormones does not necessarily last throughout life.[35] Walking may also have a major clinical role in the rehabilitation of patients, particularly the elderly, in primary care, where its scope for reducing disability and handicap could be considerable.[36]

The retention of function into old age is not just a concern for the already elderly. Some physical decline with age is inevitable, and reversing decline is much more problematic than prevention, or reducing the gradient of deterioration. For this reason the habit of regular physical activity such as walking throughout adult life, especially the middle years, will ensure that decline, when it does occur, does so from a relatively high level. This applies to bone density especially, which is less amenable to reversal than muscle strength, power and endurance.[37] Unlike other forms of physical activity, walking shows very little, if any, decline in middle age. It is a year round, readily repeatable, self reinforcing, habit forming activity and the main option for increasing physical activity in sedentary populations.[36]

The psychological benefits of physical activity are also well documented.[38,39] Research shows that those who are physically active or have higher levels of cardiorespiratory fitness have enhanced moods, higher self-esteem, greater confidence in their ability to perform tasks requiring physical activity and better cognitive functioning than sedentary people or those who are physically less fit. This includes moderate exercise programmes, involving brisk walking,[40] and may be particularly effective for treatment of depression, anxiety and other mood states.[41]

Cycling

Cycling is one of the simplest and most effective ways of getting fit, and riding to school or work means physical activity can form part of the daily routine. Cycling also enables a far greater geographical area to be accessed than can be met solely by walking. Yet in the last 50 years, cycling has changed from a mainstream mode of transport to one largely sidelined by policy makers and has declined to a

The National Travel Survey (1985/6) found that there was an 80% increase in the number of bicycles owned but only a 16% increase in cycle traffic. Despite this rise in cycle traffic, the rise in all road travel has meant the percentage of that undertaken by cycle has continued to fall.[43] The majority of cycle journeys are for commuting and business (38%) and leisure (29%)[44] and this shows that cycling is therefore a utility mode particularly important for commuting.[45]

Health benefits of cycling

In 1992, the BMA published an in-depth examination of the health risks and benefits of cycling.[43] Although it was the concern of doctors over the high levels of death and injury caused to cyclists that led to the production of the report, in the course of preparing

Figure 4
The decline in cycling[3]

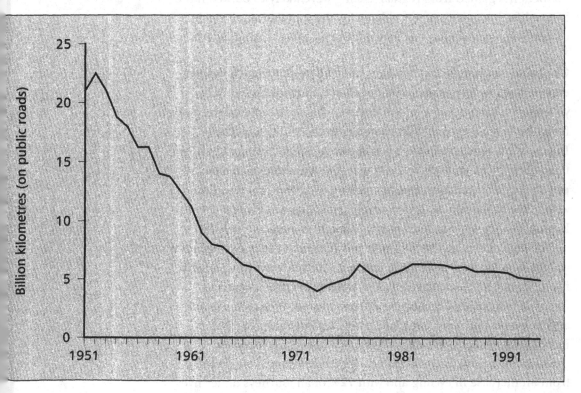

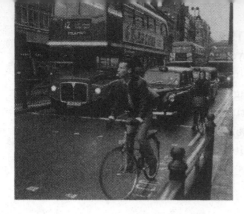

Even in the current hostile traffic environment, the benefits gained from regular cycling are likely to outweight the risk of accidents.

the document considerable evidence was found of the health benefits for regular cyclists. It was found that an increase in cycling was particularly beneficial in reducing coronary heart disease, obesity and hypertension as well as increasing overall fitness. The report also contained an estimate of the number of years of life lost through cycling accidents compared to the number of years of life gained through improved health and fitness due to regular cycling. It concluded that even in the current hostile traffic environment, the benefits gained from regular cycling were likely to outweigh the loss of life through cycling accidents for the population of regular cyclists. One calculation has shown the ratio to be around 20:1.[46]

One study, among factory workers, concluded that regular cyclists enjoy a level of fitness equivalent to that of individuals ten years younger[47] and another found that those who cycled 60 miles a week from the age of 35 could add two years to their life expectancy.[29] A Dutch study concluded that everyday or common cycling as part of normal daily activities can yield much the same improvements in physical performance as specific training programmes. For those with a low initial fitness level, a single trip distance of three kilometres per day was found to be enough to improve physical performance.[48] A small additional consideration is that cycling is not weight-bearing and, as a result, people with some forms of arthritis find it easier to cycle than walk.[49] A move away from motorized forms of transport to cycling would also lead to reductions in air and noise pollution in towns and cities and largely solve the increasing problem of traffic congestion. There are therefore considerable individual and public health benefits to be gained from an increase in cycling and with 72% of all journeys under five

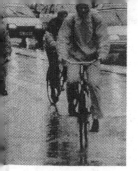

cycling to work regularly, physical activity can form part of the daily routine.

Encouraging walking and cycling

A range of recommendations have been made to promote cycling and walking, protect vulnerable road users and give more priority at every stage of the planning process for roads and transport routes to cyclists and pedestrians [42,43,50] but concerns have been expressed that encouraging cycling and walking will lead to an increase in casualties and fatalities. This is not the case however, where vulnerable road users are properly catered for. For example, by distance travelled, cycling in the Netherlands is five times safer than in Britain, and in Denmark 12 times.[51] In York, the policy of prioritising health promoting modes of transport, whilst restraining motor traffic has led to casualty reductions well above the national average (see Table 2). York has one of the largest pedestrian street networks in Europe, with a target for increasing walking related to work in the city from 13% to 14% by 2006, 22% of work related trips are already made by bicycle. Although the target increase of 1% may seem small, this must be considered in the light of the continuing decline in walking whereby maintenance of current levels is difficult.

Table 2
Changes to road casualties in York and the UK[52]
(Average percentage change 1990-94 from 1981-85)

Casualties	York (% change)	UK (% change)
All casualties	-40	-1.5
Pedestrians	-36	-15
Cyclists	-29.5	-12
Powered two wheelers	-65	-54
Car passengers	-16	+16
Car drivers	+2.5	+41.5

This table refers to road casualties only and not fatalities. Although deaths from road traffic accidents are in decline (see Table 4), there have been sharp increases in slight injuries for car users (see Chapter 4).

European countries has been analysed in order to propose effective measures for Great Britain.[50] There have been some considerable successes in increasing cycle use in some cities (see Table 3). The most successful cycle policies are those which are part of broader, sustainable transport policies. However, one specific measure which has proven to be central to improving cyclists' safety is widespread traffic calming to reduce traffic speeds.[50] In Oxfordshire a reduction of 59% of all accidents and 75% in pedestrian accidents has been achieved through traffic calming.[53] Within the UK, the introduction of a number of 20mph zones has been shown to be effective with a 60% reduction in accidents.[54]

Table 3
Successful schemes to increase cycle use in European cities[50]

City	Population	% of journeys by cycle (city centre)	Increase in cycle use (over time)	Main traffic measures
Basel	172,000	16	8-16% (1970-90)	• tram priority • traffic restraint • cycle network (city wide)
Graz	240,000	14	7-14% (1979-91)	• pedestrian measures • parking reduction • traffic calming • cycle parking & cycling
Hanover	550,000	16	9-16%	• land use planning • traffic calming • cycle routes (450km) • car parking control
Münster	280,000	43	29-43% (1981-92)	• quality cycle routes • links to public transport • traffic calming
Delft	80,000	43	40-43% (1982-85)	• compact land use • traffic cells • complete cycle network

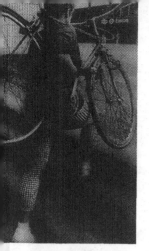

incorporating walking and cycling into a journey involving a mode of public transport, benefits health may result.

There are substantial health gains to be made by increasing walking and cycling as both primary and secondary modes of transport. As travelling by public transport is the safest of all forms of road transport, incorporating walking and cycling into a journey involving a mode of public transport could significantly increase benefits to individual and public health.[55] Given the percentage of the population for whom lack of physical activity is a risk factor for health (70% of men, 80% of women) it would seem appropriate to find means of reducing this risk, whilst also meeting other needs, ie. those of transport and access.

There are, however, barriers to walking and cycling such as lack of safe provision and fears for personal safety when in isolated areas. Individuals may opt for travel by car as this can create a feeling of personal safety and therefore reduce feelings of anxiety and stress. Individuals need to be able to make healthier transport choices through safe, appropriate and widespread provision for walking and cycling and this has been successfully achieved in parts of Great Britain and Europe. At the national level, the Department of Transport launched a National Cycling Strategy and established a National Walking Forum Steering Group in 1996. The former set a target of quadrupling the number of trips by cycle by 2012 (from 1996 baseline).[56] The latter have issued a consultation document on walking which examined the integration of walking as a proper mode of transport. The current barriers to walking were explored and questions posed as to how these could be overcome. Recommendations from the Group included the need for a national transport policy to promote walking in conjunction with local policies; create urban areas that minimise car dependency and promote walking to school. However, the document made no specific mention of setting targets for increasing levels of walking .[57] The government has also provided guidance to local authorities on the prioritization and promotion of cycling.[45]

4 **The health impact of road transport**

Introduction

Historically the main focus of concern over road transport among doctors and health care staff has been road traffic casualties since these are acute, require immediate medical treatment, and are directly attributable. The contribution of road traffic to air and noise pollution and the subsequent risk to health has become an increasing focus in the past two decades with the rapid motorization of society and growing congestion. These adverse effects, however important, may be described as being the tip of an iceberg of negative health impacts of road transport. Road traffic accidents and pollution are relatively easy to measure, whereas the health implications of reductions in walking and cycling which have accompanied rising motorization, damage to social support networks, inequality of access, for example to affordable and healthy diets, are frequently chronic, difficult to quantify, and mediated by other factors. Figure 5 illustrates the health impacts that may be attributable, in part at least, to increasing motorization. Health impacts can be divided into those where quantifiable evidence is available — the more direct effects — and to those where the evidence is more qualitative with 'predicted' health impacts — indirect effects. The evidence associated with these impacts is discussed in the following sections, alongside mechanisms for reducing adverse health impacts.

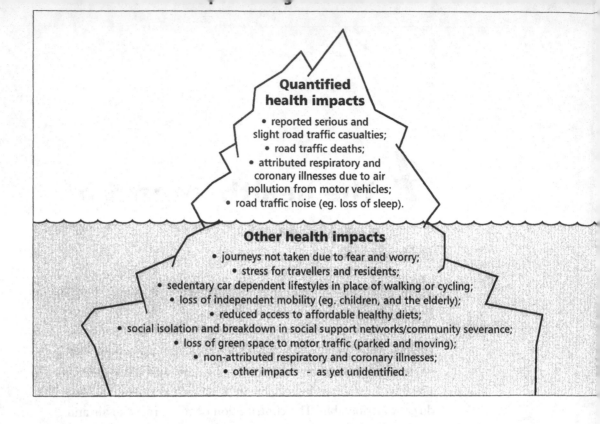

Quantified health impacts

- reported serious and slight road traffic casualties;
- road traffic deaths;
- attributed respiratory and coronary illnesses due to air pollution from motor vehicles;
- road traffic noise (eg. loss of sleep).

Other health impacts

- journeys not taken due to fear and worry;
- stress for travellers and residents;
- sedentary car dependent lifestyles in place of walking or cycling;
- loss of independent mobility (eg. children, and the elderly);
- reduced access to affordable healthy diets;
- social isolation and breakdown in social support networks/community severance;
- loss of green space to motor traffic (parked and moving);
- non-attributed respiratory and coronary illnesses;
- other impacts - as yet unidentified.

Road traffic accidents

Both the number of road deaths and reported serious injuries occurring on Britain's roads are declining. In 1996, 44,473 people were reported seriously injured and 3,598 people were killed, which is the lowest annual fatalities figure since records began in 1926. Slight injuries however, have shown a 4% increase to 272,231 people in 1996 compared to the 1995 figures. Fatalities are now 36% below the 1981-1985 average baseline and serious injuries are 40% below, whilst slight injuries are 13% above.[59,60] The general trend, therefore is that deaths and serious injuries are decreasing but slight injuries are increasing.

For pedestrians, the number of casualties for 1996 has decreased by 1% from 1995 levels to 46,381. There were 997 pedestrian deaths, a decrease of 4%, and serious injuries decreased by 6% to 10,611.[60] Compared to the 1981-1985 baseline average, pedestrian deaths

Great Britain	Rates per billion passenger kilometres					
	1981	**1986**	**1991**	**1992**	**1993**	**Average 1983-1993**
Motorcycle	115.8	100.3	94.4	97.0	94.6	102.9
Foot	76.9	75.3	62.5	58.5	56.2	68.8
Pedal cycle	56.9	49.6	46.8	43.4	41.3	48.5
Water*	0.4	0.5	0.0	0.5	0.0	9.2
Car	6.1	5.1	3.7	3.5	3.0	4.3
Van	3.8	3.8	2.2	2.2	1.7	2.6
Rail	1.0	0.9	0.8	0.4	0.4	0.9
Bus or coach	0.3	0.5	0.6	0.4	0.8	0.5
Air*	0.2	0.5	0.0	0.1	0.0	0.2

* Data are for United Kingdom

have decreased by 44% and serious injuries by 34%. Statistics also show that cyclist casualties have decreased. There were 203 cyclist deaths in 1996, a decrease of 5% on 1995 figures, slight injuries have decreased by 2% (to 24,534) and serious injuries are down 6% to 3,582.[60] Table 4 shows the passenger death rate by mode of transport as reported by the Central Statistical Office 1996.[3]

However, whilst these figures appear encouraging, it is generally accepted that there is considerable under reporting of serious and slight injuries and thus the figures could be a serious underestimation of accident rates. The Department of Transport has used the decline in deaths and serious injuries to claim that the roads are becoming safer. Yet this is highly contentious because the number of casualties is a poor measure of safety. It is true that the chances of being killed in a car have been reduced by a factor of at least five since the 1950's, largely due to vehicle design focusing on greater occupant protection but the chances of being slightly injured have risen. A better indication of safety would be to consider the most vulnerable road users, and this suggests that the overall decline in pedestrian and cyclist deaths and casualties has resulted, in Britain in 1990 only 7% of seven year olds went to school alone and 47% were taken by car[61] at an estimated cost of between £10 and £20 million annually. This compares to 1971 when 72% of seven year olds travelled to school unaccompanied.

The available data does not illustrate the true risk to pedestrians, particularly in relation to other modes of transport. Casualty rates for other modes are usually expressed per 100 million kilometres, whereas for pedestrians it is usually in terms of 100,000 population as no measures of exposure exist for walks of all lengths on different types of road. A study carried out by the AA Foundation for Road Safety, looked at exposure to risk amongst pedestrians.[65] When exposure was taken into account 411 casualties per 100 million kilometres walked was recorded as opposed to 34 per 100 million kilometres for vehicles. The study provided a number of useful insights into relative risks of different age groups, the greatly increased risk when walking in the dark, and the role of planning and environment in contributing to pedestrian casualties.

The hypothesis that walking is in fact getting more dangerous can be illustrated by considering one group —10-14 year olds — whose exposure levels as pedestrians are likely to have changed little over previous decades and are less likely to be escorted by parents than younger children. In this group the risk of being killed in road accidents nearly doubled between 1955 and 1987.[66] This was compatible with research findings from the former West Germany where child pedestrian deaths (0-15 year olds) and casualties more than doubled between 1960 and 1980.[67]

In 1987, the Department of Transport established a one third road accident casualty reduction target to be achieved by the year 2000. More recently, however, it has acknowledged concerns that an all-casualty target could lead to people being encouraged to avoid vulnerable yet health promoting forms of travel.[68] Tables 5 and 6 illustrate that being struck by a car is by far the most likely cause of death and serious injury among both pedestrians and cyclists. These statistics reveal the need to tackle the risk being posed by motor cars. The tables show that pedestrians and cyclists pose a very small risk to other categories of road user. However, concern is often expressed about 'dangerous' cycling, on pavements for example,

Colliding vehicle	Single vehicle accident (SVA)	Multiple vehicle accident	Total	%	Vehicle casualties in SVA	Pedestrian casualties over vehicle casualties
Pedal cycle	93	11	104	0.8	20	5.2
Motorcycle	381	36	417	3.4	65	6.4
Car	9,627	683	10,310	83.9	88	117.2
Bus or coach	405	19	424	3.4	10	42.4
Light goods	544	69	613	5.0	6	102.2
Heavy goods	248	43	219	2.4	5	58.2
Other	112	6	118	1.0	2	59.0
Total	11,424	869	12,293	100.0	196	62.7

Table 6
Cyclists killed, seriously injured in 1995[68]

Colliding vehicle	Two vehicle accident	Multiple (3+) vehicle accident	Total	%	Non-cyclist casualties in these accidents	Cyclist casualties over non-cyclist casualties
Pedal cycle	43	12	55	1.5	-	-
Motorcycle	63	11	74	2.1	34	2.2
Car	2,861	131	2,992	83.1	50	59.8
Bus or coach	49	3	52	1.4	3	17.3
Light goods	192	6	198	5.5	3	66.0
Heavy goods	162	11	173	4.8	5	34.6
Other	34	5	39	1.1	3	13.0
Total	3,406	194	3,600	100.0	98	36.7

Association have issued a joint statement on walking and cycling to highlight how solutions to the problems for cyclists and pedestrians are common to both parties and that the priority should be for appropriate road design and reductions in traffic speeds.[69] Shared use of pathways was viewed as a last resort and where it is the only solution, and flows of cyclists/pedestrians are high, a level of segregation should be provided.[69]

Speed

Speed has been recognised for some years to be a key determinant of road injuries and their severity.[70,71] This is supported by an international review, including evidence from the reduction of speed limits from 65 mph to 55 mph in many American States.[72] The Department of Transport calculated that driving too fast causes 77,000 injuries and approximately 1,200 road deaths a year, and ran a major speed reduction campaign, 'Kill Your Speed — Not a Child'. However, a survey of speeds driven on a variety of roads in 1995 found that seven out of ten cars and well over half of all heavy goods vehicles exceeded the limits.[73] These figures remain the same for 1996, with 72% of cars exceeding the 30 mph limit and 57% exceeding the 70 mph limit on motorways.[74] Strategies to reduce speed include driver education, traffic calming and enforced lower speed limits through the use of speed cameras, for example. It is

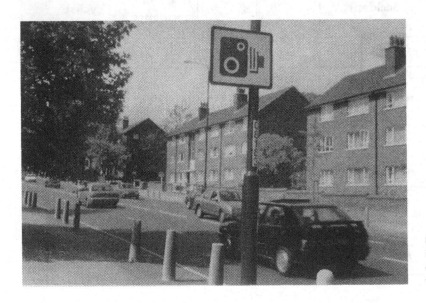

Excessive speed causes 77,000 injuries and 1,200 deaths a year — enforcement of lower speed limits is therefore essential.

particularly at risk of road traffic accidents, have been evaluated.[75] The limited evidence on educational and training interventions indicated that enhanced driver education courses had little or no effect.

Where lower speed limits have been enforced through traffic calming, the most vulnerable groups tend to gain through reduced casualties and increased independent mobility. There is a strong case for lower speed limits so that 20 mph could become the norm in built-up areas.[54] There is some evidence that while such schemes are relatively cost-effective there may be opportunities for reductions in implementation costs. In Graz, Austria, widespread introduction of 30 km/hour zones in residential areas, with minimal traffic calming, has achieved considerable success in reducing casualties.[76] Moreover, in-vehicle variable speed limiters, which respond on reaching specific speed limit zones, have been proposed as the most effective and efficient means of achieving speed reductions. If lower speed led to some reversal of the trend for longer distances being travelled, and to some people seeking to satisfy their journey purposes locally, it has been suggested that the benefits to travellers might outweigh the losses, even without taking into account the gains from reduced vehicle mileage.[77]

Alcohol

Although fatalities and casualties related to drink driving have decreased substantially within the UK (from 27,220 total casualties in 1985 to 15,160 in 1994)[78] drink driving still kills around ten people every week. However, it is not only drivers who are at risk, alcohol also contributes to pedestrian accidents. A study of pedestrian activity and risk recorded 11% of those injured as being drunk or having consumed alcohol.[65] In 1996 the BMA published a report on the effect of alcohol and other drugs on driving and made several recommendations including a reduction in the permitted blood alcohol concentration (BAC) for driving from 80mg/100ml to 50mg/100ml and the introduction of random breath testing which could lead to further reductions in accidents and injuries related to drinking and driving.[79] In addition, the provision of adequate and affordable public transport would assist in reducing the perceived need to drive after drinking.

While there are still uncertainties about the effects of some pollutants on health there is a large and growing body of scientific evidence as to the effects of the key emissions from road transport. In recent years this has been reflected by increasing concerns, both among physicians, politicians, and the public at large. While a potential hazard to the population generally, air pollution is especially a threat to vulnerable groups such as pregnant women, the elderly, people suffering from respiratory and coronary illnesses[80], children[81] and for workers with high occupational pollution exposure levels.[82,83]

Road transport emissions

Table 7 illustrates road transport's contribution to some key emissions. Emissions vary under different driving conditions so that in urban areas most pollutant concentrations are found to be higher. For example, particulate emissions from road transport rise from about 25% of total emissions nationally to over 80% in London.[84] The Government has launched a UK Air Quality Strategy with targets for reductions in eight pollutants. However, the Strategy has already been criticised on the grounds that it contains no specific targets for traffic volume, which is still set to almost double between 1994 and 2025.[13]

Table 7
Pollutant emissions from road transport in the UK: 1994[78]

Pollutant	% share of total emissions from road transport
Nitrogen oxides	53
Carbon monoxide	90
Volatile organic compounds	40
Lead	58
Black smoke	58
Particulates (PM_{10}s)	25*

*1993 figure

carcinogen, has been implicated in contributing to the total number of leukaemia deaths.[85,86] The level of emissions from individual cars is being reduced by the use of catalytic converters but there is no safe threshold level for benzene.[87] Other lesser sources of benzene include diesel exhausts and evaporation of petrol during its distribution, delivery and the refuelling of cars.

Diesel particulate in the air can aggravate respiratory diseases such as bronchitis and asthma[88] and the particulates have been classified as a probable human carcinogen.[89] There is evidence that occupational exposure among professional drivers is linked to higher risk of bladder cancer, kidney cancer and non-Hodgkin's lymphoma[90] although study samples have generally been small.[91]

Transport is also responsible for over 25% of the UK's carbon dioxide emissions, affecting the global climate, and consequently a major public health threat.[92,93]

Evidence from Europe and North America has identified that under urban driving conditions car occupants are exposed to the poorest air quality. Benzene (and other hydrocarbons), carbon monoxide, and nitrogen dioxide have been found to be substantially higher for vehicle occupants than for those outside.[94,95] This is attributed partly to occupants being 'in the road', in the line of exhaust pipes with vehicle air conditioning drawing in air from the road environment so circulating some of the most polluted air. In slow traffic or at standstill a car's air intake will be heavily contaminated by the exhaust emissions of the vehicle ahead, often only a few feet away. Other research has found that the uptake of nitrogen dioxide among cyclists has been noted to be higher than that of car drivers, with other pollutants approaching levels in cars.[96]

Particulate matter

Particulate matter refers to solid or liquid material present in the air in particles small enough to remain in suspension for hours or days. Particulate matter may therefore travel considerable distances from the source of the pollution and may vary widely in its chemical and physical characteristics. Particulate matter, especially that with an aerodynamic diameter of less than 10 μm (PM_{10}), is viewed by many times more particulates under urban driving conditions,[99] and 30-100 times more than a petrol vehicle fitted with a three way regulated catalytic converter.[100] PM_{10}s have been identified as being of most concern as this is the size likely to pass the nose and mouth. The size range of particles able to reach deeper parts of the respiratory tract are those of less than 2.5 µm in diameter ($PM_{2.5}$). Much of what is monitored as PM_{10} will in fact be less than 2.5 µm in diameter ie $PM_{2.5}$. In the United States the Environmental Protection Agency (EPA) has announced new limits to restrict $PM_{2.5}$, primarily due to a lawsuit against them by the American Lung Association over the EPA's failure to review air quality standards. In the UK, the Department of Health's Committee on the Medical Effects of Air Pollutants (COMEAP) has suggested that determination of $PM_{2.5}$ at selected sites would be valuable[101] as currently only PM_{10} is monitored.

The Government's Expert Panel on Air Quality Standards has recommended a standard of $50mg/m^3$ of PM_{10} as a running 24 hour average. Yet the Department of the Environment noted that the recommended daily standard was exceeded for about 10% of the year at most measurement sites in the UK.[97] This sits uncomfortably besides evidence that rises of $10 mg/m^3$ are accompanied by an increase in mortality of about 1% in the population, including elevated relative risk from both respiratory and cardiac causes, of around 3.4% and 1.4% respectively.[102,103] Walters has reported that death rates from heart and lung disease are up to 37% higher in cities with high levels of fine particulates.[104]

COMEAP examined in-depth the health effects of non-biological particles, PM_{10}.[101] The Committee concluded that the reported associations between daily concentrations of particles and acute effects on health principally reflected a real relationship and not some artefact of technique or the effect of some confounding factor. People with pre-existing respiratory and/or cardiac disorders are at most risk of acute effects from exposure to particles. However, the committee found no evidence that healthy individuals were likely to experience acute health effects due to UK levels of particles. By contrast, the most carefully conducted study of the link between long term exposure to air pollution and mortality found air pollution to be positively associated with death from lung cancer considered this study and other evidence and concluded that it would be 'prudent' to consider the association between particulates and chronic health effects as causal.

Asthma and air pollution

There has been an increase of about 50% in the prevalence of childhood asthma over the last 30 years and data from the Department of Health reveals that hospital admissions for the condition have increased from 4,000 in 1980 to 10,000 in 1990.[106] It has been suggested that these trends are related to air pollution with the proposal that air pollution could both initiate asthma in previously healthy individuals or aggravate or provoke symptoms in those already asthmatic. In a number of studies, correlations between neighbourhood traffic volumes and child respiratory symptoms have been reported, including hospital admissions for

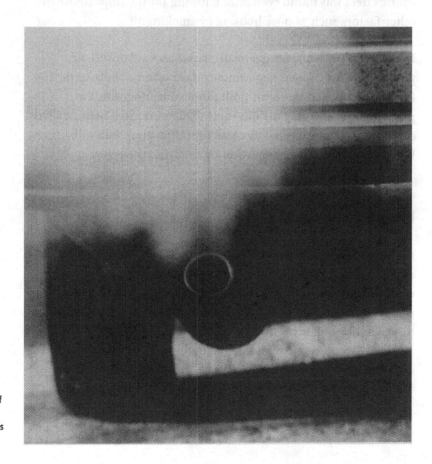

...hicle exhaust contains a number of
...llutants and can aggravate
...spiratory diseases such as bronchitis
...d asthma.

chronic respiratory symptoms among children living along streets with high traffic density, and mild dyspnoea more prevalent among adults.[109] COMEAP has reviewed the available evidence to determine whether asthma and outdoor air pollution are in fact linked.[110] The Committee concluded that the available evidence did not support a causative role for outdoor air pollution. In relation to worsening or provocation of symptoms it was concluded that only a small proportion of patients may experience a clinically significant effect.

There may also be a link between perceived air quality and psychosomatic symptoms which have been associated with recurrent colds and chronic bronchitis, including among school children.[111] A study conducted in Scotland and the North of England examined a range of general symptoms in relation to traffic levels. For symptoms such as sore eyes and dry cough a clear and quantifiable traffic effect was found even after allowing for the importance of other factors such as poor housing or smoking.[112]

Despite the evidence for the health risks associated with air pollution, Government departments have taken a short-term view (ten years) of road traffic air pollution, coinciding with the predicted decline in emissions up to 2005 associated with catalytic converters. The projected increase in traffic after 2005 will, however, negate the benefits won by catalytic converters.

Noise pollution

Although noise has become widespread in modern society the exact extent is not well quantified. *The Health of the Nation*[1] discussion document on including the 'environment' as a sixth key area noted that less than 1% of the population of England and Wales is thought to be exposed to an average noise above 65 dB(A) at night although around 10% of the population is thought to be exposed to noise above this level during the day.[113]

Traffic noise is a widespread form of noise disturbance, affecting sleep and mental health. Sleep interference is probably the most important effect in terms of human health and wellbeing after long-term exposure.[114] Up to 63% of dwellings are exposed to a level of night-time noise high enough to interfere with sleep.[115] Sleep quality decreases with increased number of noise events at 60 dB(A),[116] while road traffic noise during the first hours of sleep tends to disturb sleep more than when it occurs later in the night. The main effect of exposure is a reduction in the total amount of rapid eye movement (REM) sleep and an increased duration of intermittent waking during hours of exposure.[117]

Intermittent traffic noise may decrease time spent in slow-wave sleep (SWS). In urban areas large numbers of young adults may be chronically deprived of SWS, mood states may be affected, and minor effects on heart rate may occur after many years of nightly exposure to noise.[118] Noise may also have important psycho-social effects with evidence for depression among people exposed to high levels of traffic noise.[119]

Traffic noise is estimated to be at 80 dB(A) in a busy street and 100 dB(A) for a heavy lorry 7m away[120] and it is generally accepted that regular, long term exposure to such noise could result in noise induced hearing loss. Noise pollution has been shown to have significant effects on concentration, stress and increases in blood pressure with an increasing likelihood of aggression being shown.[121] Overall, traffic noise can reduce perceived environmental quality, increase sleeping problems and health worries which may lead to recourse to health services.[122]

There is at present no provision for noise checks as part of the vehicle test (MoT), and no measures are planned under the Environmental Health Action Plan to address road traffic noise, either through engine and exhaust noise or tyre noise reduction programmes.[123] The latter may be particularly affected by reduced speeds.

Social support has been proposed as either directly promoting health and health behaviours or as buffering the adverse effect of stressors.[124] Low levels of social support have been linked to increased mortality rates from all causes to the extent that people with few social contacts may be at more than twice the risk of those with many contacts.[125] Other research has corroborated this and also suggests that good social support networks are most important for vulnerable groups such as the elderly[126,127,128] and children.[129] A review of the role of psychosocial stress and social support concluded that both had an influence on coronary heart disease, social support more so than stress. Lack of social support increased mortality from coronary heart disease up to four times.[130]

Community severance through road building has been defined as 'the sum of the divisive effects a road has on those in the locality'.[131] Most research has been to assess the effects of increases in traffic, either over time with traffic growth or as a result of the building of a new road and human adaptations to these changes.[132] Appleyard and Lintell's classic study of the impact of traffic on three similar streets in an area of San Francisco helps to illustrate how traffic volumes and speed affects street use for non-traffic functions (see Figures 6-9).[133] They observed behaviour in relation to differing levels of traffic, using a range of environmental indicators, in order to interpret the 'livability' of streets. These included: pedestrian delay times, counts of street activities, closed windows, drawn blinds, parked cars, litter, flower boxes, and other signs of personal care.

Three streets were studied, similar in all aspects except traffic volume, so that one street had 2,000 vehicles per day (Light street), another 8,000 (Moderate street), and the third 16,000 vehicles per day (Heavy street). All aspects of perceived 'livability' were examined; absence of noise, stress, pollution, levels of social interaction, territorial extent, environmental awareness and safety. These were all found to correlate inversely with traffic density. Safety, for example, was perceived to be less of a problem on the Light street than the others.

Residents were asked how many friends and acquaintances they had on their street. On Light street the number of friends was three

San Francisco: Traffic hazard on three streets[133]

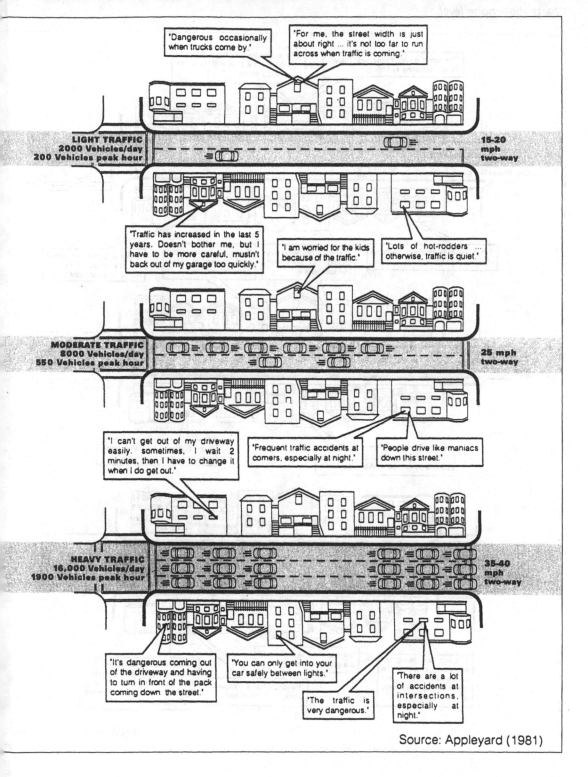

Source: Appleyard (1981)

San Francisco: Noise, stress and pollution on three streets[133]

Charts show noise level.

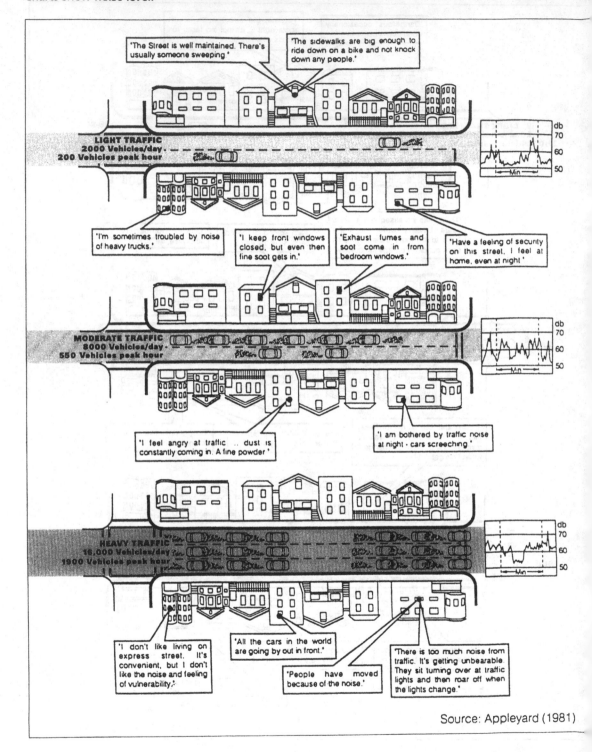

'The Street is well maintained. There's usually someone sweeping.'

'The sidewalks are big enough to ride down on a bike and not knock down any people.'

LIGHT TRAFFIC
2000 Vehicles/day
200 Vehicles peak hour

'I'm sometimes troubled by noise of heavy trucks.'

'I keep front windows closed, but even then fine soot gets in.'

'Exhaust fumes and soot come in from bedroom windows.'

'Have a feeling of security on this street. I feel at home, even at night.'

MODERATE TRAFFIC
8000 Vehicles/day
550 Vehicles peak hour

'I feel angry at traffic .. dust is constantly coming in. A fine powder.'

'I am bothered by traffic noise at night - cars screeching.'

HEAVY TRAFFIC
16,000 Vehicles/day
1900 Vehicles peak hour

'I don't like living on express street. It's convenient, but I don't like the noise and feeling of vulnerability.'

'All the cars in the world are going by out in front.'

'People have moved because of the noise.'

'There is too much noise from traffic. It's getting unbearable. They sit turning over at traffic lights and then roar off when the lights change.'

Source: Appleyard (1981)

San Francisco: Home territory on three streets[133]

...ines show where they had friends or acquaintances. Small dots show where people are said to gather.

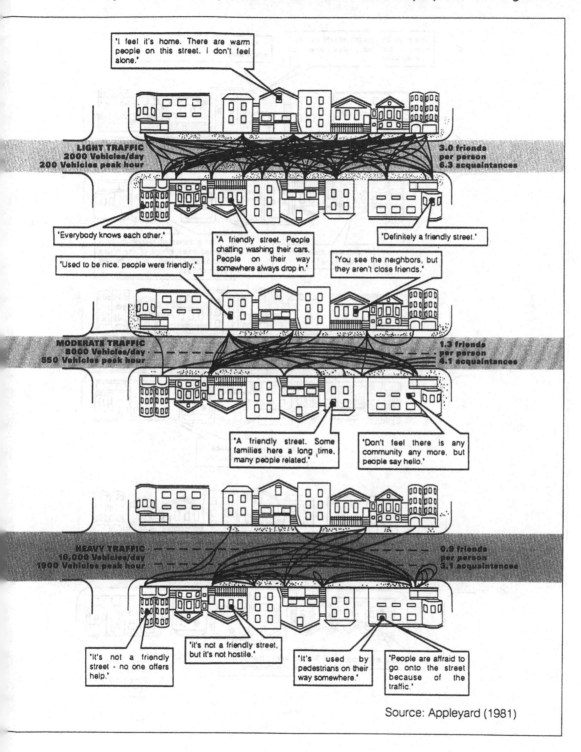

'I feel it's home. There are warm people on this street. I don't feel alone.'

LIGHT TRAFFIC
2000 Vehicles/day
200 Vehicles peak hour

3.0 friends
per person
6.3 acquaintances

'Everybody knows each other.'

'Used to be nice. people were friendly.'

'A friendly street. People chatting washing their cars. People on their way somewhere always drop in.'

'Definitely a friendly street.'

'You see the neighbors, but they aren't close friends.'

MODERATE TRAFFIC
8000 Vehicles/day
550 Vehicles peak hour

1.3 friends
per person
4.1 acquaintances

'A friendly street. Some families here a long time, many people related.'

'Don't feel there is any community any more, but people say hello.'

HEAVY TRAFFIC
16,000 Vehicles/day
1900 Vehicles peak hour

0.9 friends
per person
3.1 acquaintances

'It's not a friendly street - no one offers help.'

'it's not a friendly street, but it's not hostile.'

'It's used by pedestrians on their way somewhere.'

'People are afraid to go onto the street because of the traffic.'

Source: Appleyard (1981)

San Francisco: Home territory on three streets[133]

Lines show areas people indicated as their 'home territory'.

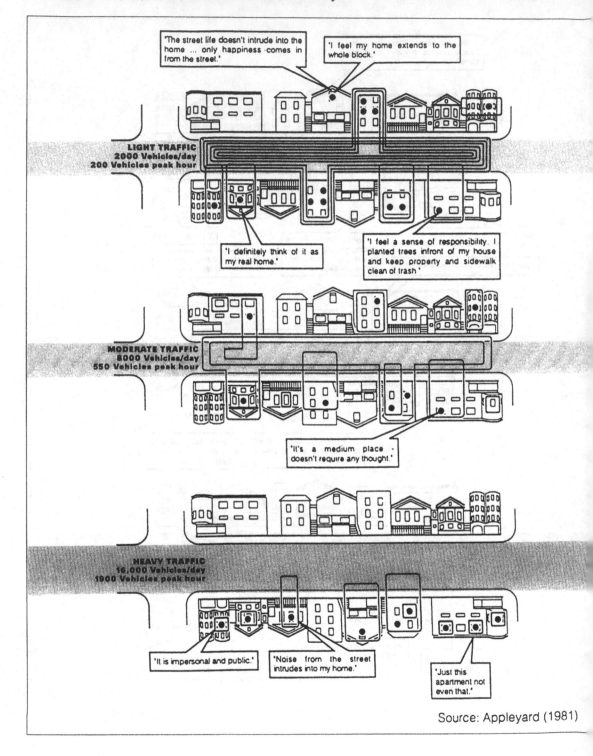

'The street life doesn't intrude into the home ... only happiness comes in from the street.'

'I feel my home extends to the whole block.'

LIGHT TRAFFIC
2000 Vehicles/day
200 Vehicles peak hour

'I definitely think of it as my real home.'

'I feel a sense of responsibility. I planted trees infront of my house and keep property and sidewalk clean of trash.'

MODERATE TRAFFIC
8000 Vehicles/day
550 Vehicles peak hour

'It's a medium place - doesn't require any thought.'

HEAVY TRAFFIC
16,000 Vehicles/day
1900 Vehicles peak hour

'It is impersonal and public.'

'Noise from the street intrudes into my home.'

'Just this apartment not even that.'

Source: Appleyard (1981)

families with children felt relatively free from traffic dangers. In contrast, Heavy street had little or no pavement activity and was used 'solely as a corridor between the sanctuary of individual homes and the outside world'. Appleyard and Lintell found that decline of environmental quality on Heavy street had led to a process of environmental selection and adaptation in the street's residential make-up which had changed significantly over the years as a result of the hostile traffic environment. Residents kept very much to themselves and had withdrawn from the street environment. As such there was little sense of community. Most families with children had departed from Heavy street, although some elderly people, finding it too costly or too much effort to move, became 'locked in'. Some were sleeping in back bedrooms to reduce traffic noise disturbance. Moderate traffic street fell half way between the two.

Impact of traffic on neighbourhoods

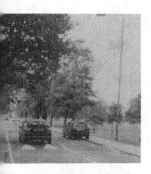

affic calming schemes can lead improvements in quality of life r local residents and improved fety for pedestrians and clists.

More recent studies have also assessed the impact of traffic on neighbourhoods and have shown that related to traffic volume, air and noise pollution are viewed as serious problems. A study of the environmental impacts of traffic in Oslo[134] noted that both the elderly and families with young children stress that road traffic results in insecurity, and make it difficult for pedestrians and cyclists to get around. In Edinburgh a study of the severance effects on pedestrians also found significant delays for the young and the elderly in crossing roads, with the latter being many more times disadvantaged than younger adults.[135] Conversely, where lower speeds are engineered through traffic calming, evidence suggests some perceived improvements in quality of life or 'livability', including improved safety for pedestrians and cyclists,[136] benefits for families with children,[137] and greater independent mobility for children, especially for 7-9 year olds.[138]

Social support networks

The impact of traffic on non-traffic functions of streets is important because it can influence social support networks. While motorized transport has enabled access to friends as well as work opportunities further away than otherwise might be possible, the health 'costs' are health promoting facilities for those on foot or travelling by bicycle, including shops, health facilities, parks, and friends. The old and the young are likely to be least able to cope with such danger and either curtail activities themselves or in the case of children, are restricted by their parents.

Personal safety

Perceived danger of travel

Personal safety fears appear to have increased significantly in recent years and this has had a detrimental effect on both walking and cycling as primary and secondary modes of transport. In a recent survey by the Pedestrians' Association, 37% of pedestrians interviewed said that the largest problem they had experienced whilst walking in their local area was too much traffic. Busy roads can be intimidating to pedestrians, especially children, the disabled, elderly and those with impaired mobility.[55] A perceived danger of travel causes feelings of anxiety and pedestrians are more exposed to accidental injury, pollution noise and stress. The perceived danger of travel may also cause people to restrict their travel with a consequent loss of any health benefits that they might otherwise have gained. Fear for personal safety, especially at night, has also become an important deterrent to the use of public transport among women and the elderly.[139,140] Problems arise due to poor lighting, isolated facilities, poor visibility and lack of surveillance in subways.

Children's freedom

Many parents now feel obliged to constrain the activities of their children in order to safeguard them from road traffic,[141] and one of the biggest social changes in childhood recently has been the unwillingness of most parents to allow their children to walk or cycle to school for fear of accidents and assaults. In Britain, in 1990, only 7% of seven year olds went to school alone compared to 72% in 1971. For English school children, in 1990, 35% travelled to school by car compared to 10% in 1971[61] (see Figure 10).

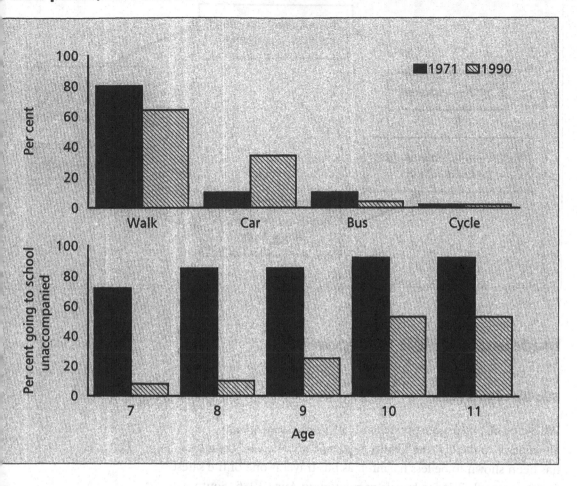

Fears about the risk of abduction or assault, often referred to as
'stranger danger', have also risen sharply in recent years and the
natural response of parents, faced with the twin dangers from traffic
and from possible assailants, has been to restrict children's freedom
of movement beyond the home, and to reduce independent
mobility. This is likely, however, to have a serious effect on the
physical health and mental development of children, as well as
depriving them of freedoms enjoyed by previous generations.[142]
Figure 11 below shows the effect of ever increasing traffic on
children's freedom of movement.

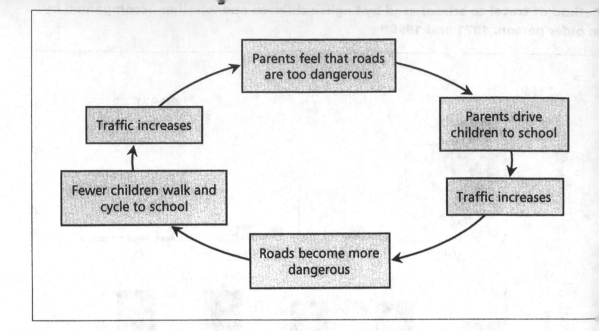

Inadequate public transport

Bus de-regulation

Where public transport provides an affordable and reliable alternative to the car, the health impact of travel on communities has been shown to be less harmful, as bus travel is one of the safest forms of travel. Prior to bus de-regulation in April 1986, South Yorkshire had one of the most comprehensive and cheap public transport systems in the UK, having frozen fares in 1975. There was a large decrease in fare prices in real terms over a ten year period, and increases in bus patronage relative to other metropolitan counties during the early 1980s resulted in an actual increase in distance travelled by bus. The public transport subsidy benefited the health of the local population by providing the social amenity of additional travel, at the least additional health cost.[143]

After de-regulation when bus fares rose by 250% in West Yorkshire, the unemployed and the retired reduced their bus journeys by over 62% and 60% respectively compared with 37% reductions for those in work and 48% reductions for school children. Research into the

women's ability to get out of the house to reach basic services, making journeys 'traumatic'. Some women found themselves isolated because levels of public transport provision did not enable them to visit their friends and relatives, reducing feelings of freedom, self-sufficiency and independence.[144] Additionally, social support networks suffered as journeys to undertake informal caring roles were more difficult to make. Subsequent increases in requests for statutory support services including home helps were recorded.[145] Moreover, the West Yorkshire research demonstrated that gender and income inequalities have a major effect on women's experience of transport. The researchers concluded that, in particular, the impact of the lack of sufficient public transport for women's health should be of much greater concern for society.[144]

Table 8 illustrates the overall sharp decline in local bus passenger journeys between 1983 and 1993-94. Although metropolitan areas

Table 8
Local bus services: passenger journeys by area 1993-94 compared with 1983[146]

	1983 (million)	1993-94 (million)	Change (%)
London	1087	1117	+2.7
English Metropolitan Area	2011	1334	-33.7
English Shire Counties	1629	1268	-22.2
England	4727	3719	-21.3
Scotland	680	526	-22.6
Wales	180	130	-27.8
Great Britain	5587	4375	-21.7
All outside London	4500	3258	-27.6

requirements, that have been disproportionately affected. Local authority franchised services are prohibitively expensive, leaving the car as a cheaper and more convenient option, while private operators view rural services as unprofitable. For community and voluntary transport provision, research has found that socio-economic variables such as car ownership, numbers of elderly, disabled people or population density do not have any significant impact on the levels of such provision, whereas larger, more populated parishes were more likely to have such schemes.[147] Car ownership, which is higher in the countryside than in urban areas, is paradoxically serving to heighten the isolation of a significant number of 'mobility disadvantaged' people.

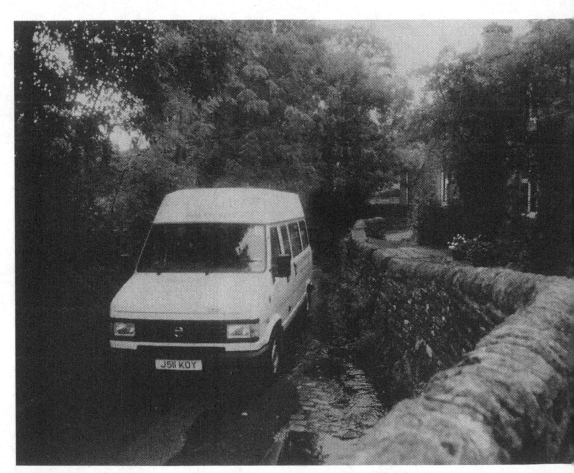

Moorlands Community Minibus, Staffordshire. Declining levels of public transport services means that community schemes become more important, especially to rural residents.

Changing patterns of food shopping

Land use planning has contributed to habitual car use for increasing types of trips. A prime example of this is reflected in changing patterns of food shopping. Total distance travelled for food shopping increased by 60% between 1975/76 and 1989/91, and miles travelled by car drivers during the same period more than doubled. Pedestrian and public transport mileage for shopping has changed little. This increased use of cars for food shopping has been a response to the growth of out of town and edge of town food and retail stores. These stores offer a large range of cheap foods, attractive to households with a car, adequate cash flow and storage facilities, who can drive to the stores and bulk buy. High income households and those with access to a car spend 79% and 73% respectively of their expenditure on food in supermarkets compared to 62% among pensioners and 60% among households with no car.[3] Indeed, some supermarkets claim that 'new sites are located where safe and convenient access is obtainable by car', and that 'today we would not open a store which did not have a large surface level car park'.[148] There is also an additional issue of where the perceived need for private motor transport has a negative impact on total household expenditure in low income households to the extent that savings may be sought in food expenditure before the car is sold. This may be particularly so for those living in rural areas.[149]

Socio-economic factors

Diseases where poor nutrition has been described as a risk factor, are more common among low income groups than among the more affluent. There is an inverse correlation between the consumption of leafy green-yellow vegetables and cardiovascular diseases and cancers, yet low income families' consumption of fruit and vegetables has nearly halved while general consumption of items such as milk, fish, meat, eggs, bread, has declined, more so in the larger poorer family.[150] Research shows that low income groups are equally well informed about, and motivated to adopt, healthy eating habits as the rest of the population, yet tend to eat a diet higher in fat, sugar and salt, and lower in fibre-rich starchy foods, vitamins been forced to increase price and reduce range of stock in order to compete. The cost of shopping at local corner stores has been found to be up to 60% higher than shopping at major stores, equivalent to £10-20 a week for an average pensioner couple.[151] Poor consumers trying to eat healthily have to choose between price or nutritious food which effectively gives them no choice.[152] This is increasingly polarising society between consumers who can and can not afford healthy diets.

Some doctors have objected to the opening of new retail developments on the grounds that they increase health inequalities, reduce availability while increasing costs of healthy diets in local shops, and increase dependence on the car, which in turn, disrupts social support networks among those already disadvantaged most.[153] The Government's own guidance to Local Authorities also supports promotion of existing urban and suburban and rural centres which are more likely to offer a choice of access, particularly for those without the use of a private car.[14]

Inequalities and transport

As with health inequalities generally,[154,155,156] the disadvantages of travel fall disproportionately on lower socio-economic groups and ethnic minorities. Health benefits are mainly experienced by people travelling by the most health promoting modes (walking and cycling), however these vulnerable groups suffer the most disadvantages imposed by motorised transport. Disadvantages are also experienced by society generally and particularly those in close proximity to those travelling. In addition, specific groups such as children, the elderly and women may be particularly adversely affected by current transport policy.

Income

Household car ownership is highly dependent on household income, (see Table 9). More men than women own cars, at 64% and 35% respectively, but ownership among women has risen far more sharply in recent years than for men (see Table 10).

	Percentage
Professional	5
Managerial	4
Intermediate non-manual	15
Junior non-manual	28
Skilled manual	14
Semi-skilled manual	33
Unskilled manual	45
Economically inactive	55

Table 10
Percentage of car ownership by gender[8]

	Male %	Female %
1992-1994	64	35
1985-1986	59	24
1975-1976	51	13

A sharp rise in car ownership among the young and those over 65 has also occurred.[8] Those over 65 are, however, less likely to have access to a car than those under 65, particularly if they live alone. For 65-74 year olds living alone 29% have access to a car. This drops to 15% for those aged 75 years and upwards.[157] An important factor in influencing mode of transport used is also multiple car ownership in households. For children's travel there is a particularly strong association. Of the 21% of children aged 5-10 years who live in a household without a car, 87% travel to school by foot, this drops sharply as car ownership in households rise. Of children living in households with two or more cars, 53% are taken to school by car, while 36% walk. There is a similar pattern for children aged 11-15

Low income households are more likely to be reliant on public transport and to have suffered most from the effects of bus de-regulation in 1986. It is likely to have made caring responsibilities and social support more difficult, including provision of child care, involving increased complexity in individual household scheduling. Low income households suffer particularly from communication deprivation in terms of information about public transport availability,[158] and women as carers have greater difficulties in accessing health services.[144] Moreover, where communities perceive access to medical care to be poor there are higher rates for hospitalisation from chronic diseases.[159] Relocation of hospital and other health care facilities to edge of town sites, poorly served by public transport, favour car users as opposed to those without access to a car. Access to healthcare facilities is also of difficulty for those in rural or isolated areas. For disabled people problems are compounded with access to health services being denied because of woefully inadequate transport provision.[160]

Socio-economic factors

Socio-economic inequalities in child injury rates increased between 1981-91, and if these gradients continue, *The Health of the Nation's*[1] accident target is not likely to be met for children in manual social classes.[161] Currently, the child pedestrian death rates for Social Class V is almost five times that of children in Social Class I. This differential in accident and injury rates has also been associated with levels of car ownership. Children from families without a car have been noted to cross a greater numbers of roads than those from car owning households. Children from households with two or more cars cross least roads as pedestrians.[162] The proportion of vehicles exceeding speed limits in low socio-economic areas is also higher than in more affluent areas[163] with higher traffic volumes,[164] despite lower car ownership.

The elderly

The current transport system is largely hostile to elderly people. Roads are often perceived as barriers to the day to day movements volumes rise.[135] Road traffic can lead to a perceived danger of travel which causes feelings of insecurity, anxiety and stress. This could in turn lead them to restrict their travel with a consequent loss of any health benefit that might otherwise have been gained. The study by Appleyard and Lintell in San Francisco (see pages 38-43) showed that with increasing volumes of traffic, elderly people found it too costly or too much effort to move and became 'locked in' and isolated.[133]

The decline in public transport services has also had a detrimental effect on the independent mobility of elderly people. Research into the effects of bus de-regulation in West Yorkshire found that reductions in bus frequencies had particularly negative effects on elderly women's ability to get out of the house to reach basic services, making journeys 'traumatic'. Some women found themselves isolated because levels of public transport provision did not enable them to visit their friends and relatives, reducing feelings of freedom, self-sufficiency and independence, [144] especially so for those in rural areas.

Children

Bagley found that children living in an environment marked by multiple social disadvantage are likely to 'acquire vulnerable characteristics, such as impulsivity and poor cognitive skills in relation to their environment, from circumstances relating to family background, including the perinatal environment'.[165] Yet it appears likely that the willingness or ability to advocate for child safety varies inversely with the need for it, mirroring Tudor Hart's inverse care law for medical care.[166] However, the need for environmental modification by which children can regain some of their 'lost' freedoms, particularly through the control and reduction of private car use is gaining ground.[167,168]

Children's needs in terms of transport policy are an area of neglect and their independent mobility and access are severely restricted by contemporary urban environments.[169,170] Children are a particularly vulnerable group as demonstrated by the high levels of casualties and deaths in childhood due to road traffic accidents. If planning of the urban environment focussed on children's needs, this would not

Accidents

Accidents are the commonest cause of hospital admissions for children between ages 5-16 in the UK. Of these admissions traffic injuries feature most prominently and in the UK death rates for child pedestrians are the second highest in Europe.[171] A recent study of trends in child mortality from unintentional injury between 1985 and 1992 concluded that if trends in child mortality from injury continued, the government target to reduce the rate by 33% by the year 2005 would not be achieved. It is likely that casualties would be higher but for the fact that parents have perceived the danger, consequently increasing restrictions on their children's independent mobility,[61,172] which could lead to serious implications for the personal development of young people. These changing travel patterns and the associated decline in children's physical activity could exact a considerable price in terms of future health problems.[64]

Where environmental changes have been made to the road environment the evidence is that children are major beneficiaries. A review of the impact of the introduction of 200 20 mph zones found reductions in child pedestrian accidents of 70%, child cyclist accidents by 48%, and overall accidents by around 60%. Significantly there was a 6.2% reduction in accidents for each 1 mph reduction in vehicle speed.[54]

Physical activity

Research suggests that mirroring adult reductions in physical activity,[20] levels of physical activity among children are declining.[173,174,175] One survey noted that 'many of today's children lack stamina; are short of breath after the simplest of exercise; have poor posture leading to lower back pain; are not interested in exercise or sport; are tired and lethargic... and seem reluctant to walk anywhere'.[176] As has been widely noted, because cardiovascular risk factors, including obesity, and unfavourable lipid profiles, tend to track from childhood to adulthood, establishing physical activity patterns in childhood is a key to reducing adult cardiovascular is therefore likely to have damaging consequences for both the health and transport sectors in the longer term through the development of habitual car use.

Independence

Beyond physical activity, the development of sensory, motor, emotional and cognitive skills takes place most fully in the form of play. Moreover, independent mobility is important in promoting self-esteem, a strong sense of identity, creative use of one's own mind and the capacity to take responsibility for oneself.[180,181] Sleap and Warburton reported that the conditions of modern society appear to inhibit children from physically active lifestyles.[175] This view is corroborated by work with 9-11 and 13-14 year olds in Birmingham which found that children themselves perceive that their ability to lead healthy lives is significantly constrained. Fear of motor traffic was a key determinant of the options they perceived to be available to them in decisions about local travel choices, and about play.[169,170] Hillman et al[61] stated that a decline in children's personal independence has three adverse consequences:

- children are denied the basic right to get around on their own;

- parents have to spend more time escorting their children;

- playing in the street, a traditional social and recreational activity is forbidden to many.

Reviews have been carried out to identify effective measures to prevent unintentional injuries in children.[182] With regard to road injuries it has been concluded that 'policy makers need to recognise the impact that broad land use and transport policies have on childhood unintentional injury and act accordingly'. For educational initiatives aimed at children there was reasonable evidence for behavioural change through education aimed at the child and or parent. It was suggested that parents needed to be involved in training programmes together with their children and that lack of co-ordination between agencies had led to fragmented road safety education in the past. However, it was emphasised that a combination of educational, environmental and legislative approaches achieved the greatest success.

Approximately 10% of the population has some degree of temporary or permanent mobility restriction at any one time. It is important, therefore, that disabled people should have the same access to the full range of transport options as everyone else and be able to use them with ease and confidence in obtaining equality and independence in society.

Access

Some people may have access to a car to help mobility, but in London 55% of disabled people do not have such access.[160] Disabled people should have full access to public transport if reduced reliance on the motor car is to be encouraged. Accessible local shops, libraries, civic amenities as well as transport systems are important in promoting good social support networks particularly among vulnerable sections of the population. This includes journeys to work. A fully accessible public transport system must also be properly integrated with other forms of transport (eg. specialised services such as dial-a-ride) and must be part of a wider accessible planning policy. There is considerable evidence to show the intrinsic benefit to the health of mobility-impaired people of an increase in their transport options. Additionally, there are demonstrable cross-sector benefits that accrue to society when such people become less in need of domiciliary services, become less benefit dependent when they are able to pursue training and eventually job opportunities, and generally are empowered to play a fuller part in society. A study of the potential for cross-sector benefits of accessible public transport systems for disabled people estimated a low value of £256 million and a potential high value of £1,161 million (1990/91).[183] Estimates were based on such factors as reduced costs for home chiropody visits and meal delivery services in addition to the potential for taking up employment.

In order to provide better access to buses the Disabled Person's Transport Advisory Committee recommends that improvements be made to the design of buses.[184] These may transpire as a result of the Disability Discrimination Act (1995) which makes it unlawful for service providers to refuse to serve a disabled person or make it difficult or impossible for a disabled person to use a service, qualified by a test of 'reasonableness'. The Act empowers the Secretary of State for the Environment, Transport and the Regions

transport, such as taxis, could become generally more accessible in a fairly short period of time. Other modes, however, such as the London Underground, will take many years to be fully converted. To be fully effective, the changes to the physical accessibility of transport vehicles need to be accompanied by comprehensive programmes of training. At the service delivery end, bus drivers, bookings clerks and other front line staff need to be helped towards a greater understanding of the different and varied needs of disabled people. Travel training for staff may also benefit mobility-impaired people, such as those with learning difficulties, who may aspire to independent use of public transport in the future.

Safety

Safety is also a key issue. A survey of visually-impaired independent travellers found that they had more accidents whilst using public transport and when walking than sighted people.[185] Virtually all respondents reported having had at least one accident whilst out walking, and over half sustained injuries. Visually-impaired pedestrians also had more accidents when crossing roads than sighted people. A number of measures were proposed to improve safety such as tactile surfaces to warn of steps and pavement edges, and improved training of bus drivers in disability awareness. To improve information and therefore remedial measures it was also proposed that public transport operators should record disability information on accident records kept for insurance purposes.

Urban and Rural inequalities

The Rural Development Commission has highlighted two key issues that can disadvantage rural residents: the high cost of car dependence; and the low and declining levels of public transport.[186] Many studies have highlighted the necessity of car ownership in rural areas and the general pattern is that car ownership is much higher in rural than urban areas as people in peripheral areas often have little or no choice but to use the car.[141] High levels of car ownership in rural areas, taken by some to reflect wealth, may instead indicate an extra burden for those on low incomes and any attempt to increase fuel taxes will have little or no effect on traffic volumes.[141]

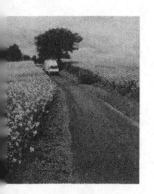

ople living in rural areas are reasingly dependent on torized transport.

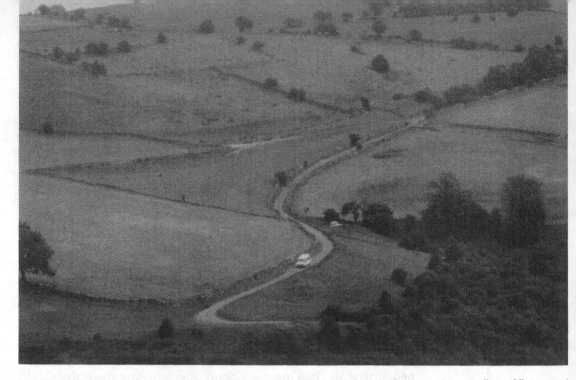

Many people living in rural areas, especially the elderly, are reliant upon community and voluntary services as well as public transport.

Levels of public transport services in rural areas are declining and with this brings a decline in beneficial modes of transport such as walking and cycling as most people will turn to the motor car as the main alternative. A significant majority of rural residents are recognised as being particularly dependent on public transport provision, including many women and elderly and young people[186] which further exacerbates inequalities. Community and voluntary transport has an important role to play as a means of meeting the needs of rural inhabitants.

In 1993, the Department of Transport introduced the 'Transport Policies and Programmes Package bids' scheme. Under this scheme, local authorities bid for funds to implement a variety of transport measures which are assessed as an integrated package. In the first two years of the scheme, the most popular measures have included priority bus schemes, cycling schemes and traffic calming measures. To date however, the package bids have been mainly aimed at relieving congestion in urban locations and rural bids have been concerned with the control of tourist-based traffic in National Parks.

result in a more strategic approach to community and voluntary transport which would benefit rural inhabitants.

Very few community or transport schemes have been found to be able to cover their costs and the funding from both the Rural Transport Development Fund (RTDF) and local authorities is critical in sustaining these schemes. There are however, concerns that new schemes are being affected by the pressure on local authority budgets and it has been recommended that the funding criteria for the RTDF should be reviewed to give a two-tier approach adopted to provide higher levels of assistance to areas with lower population densities.[147]

Although urban residents have better access to public transport services, studies show that pedestrian casualty rates are several times higher in the most urban counties than in the rural ones[55] and urban pedestrians are more likely to suffer from adverse health effects such as noise, pollution, congestion, stress and severance of communities. There are therefore different considerations to be taken into account in transport planning in rural and urban areas.

Summary

The increasing motorization of the transport system has provided benefits for some but generally at the expense of others leading to an inequitable transport system. The adverse effects of road transport policies are far broader than the obvious factors of pollution and road accidents. All factors need to be taken into account in developing an integrated sustainable and healthy transport policy.

Land use planning favouring out of town cheaper shopping and other facilities such as health and leisure primarily necessitate car use. However, people who have planned their lives around the availability of good personal transport and who live in communities where shopping, leisure and public services have been located in relation to this assumption, may suffer serious problems when sickness or frailty make them unable to use their car. Whilst some of

There are ways in which some of these negative impacts of transport policy can be addressed such as reducing traffic speeds and addressing land use planning, with the emphasis on accessibility by less damaging and safer transport modes. The chapters that follow expand on these strategies with the emphasis not only on reducing health risks but also promoting health benefits.

5 Reducing health risks and increasing health benefits through transport policy

The 'positive-negative' of car use

Many would argue that the motor car has been one of the principal instruments in the improvement of quality of life for humankind. It has the potential to fulfill many of the individual requirements for a 'good lifestyle' as defined within western society — speed, pleasure, access, individualism and personal identity[121] and the use of cars can not be considered solely as a calculated matter of costs and times.[6] However, car drivers have free access to roads and the atmosphere and this imposes costs on others that they do not bear themselves. Everyone has the same claim and the same rights to road space and access so that in the end all of the positive aspects of private motoring become negatives,[121] to a point where supply can no

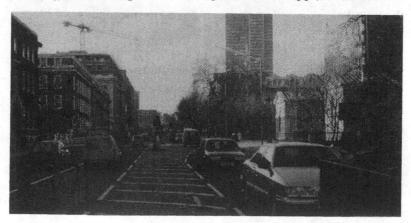

Urban driving is becoming increasingly stressful.

to other forms of transport, it is inevitable that the transport sector will continue to impose large and growing costs on the natural environment, human health and the competitiveness of the British economy.[141]

Changing attitudes

Evidence suggests that reliance on cars will not disappear and some journeys are undoubtedly necessary so policy needs to focus primarily on unnecessary car journeys, which can be attracted to other modes of transport by suitable combinations of improvement and restraint.[6] At the same time, more long term measures such as land use incentives, price signals and policy coherence would be necessary to have substantial effects on the underlying structural reasons for car dependence.[6] If cars were cheaper to buy and own but more expensive to use, this would enable more people to own cars for use when essential, but encourage all of them to use other modes of travel wherever possible.[55]

A report by the RAC[6] suggests that a significant proportion of people, perhaps a quarter to a third, would like to travel less by car if circumstances allowed. This is perhaps enhanced by the fact that motor transport is becoming increasingly stressful, and measurements of heart rate and blood pressure whilst driving have shown them to rise in congested traffic.[55] This is further supported by the 1993 British Social Attitudes Survey conducted by Social and Community Planning Research which showed that the majority of the population agreed on the need to reduce the amount of motorized traffic (see Table 11).

A comparison between societies that encourage cycling and those that do not suggests that the decisions people make about transport are not related to income, technology or the degree of urban development but to enlightened public policy and strong government support.[187] This underlies the importance of distinguishing between car dependent people and car dependent trips in any consideration of the potential impacts of changing circumstances or policies.[6]

	Percentages			
	Agree	Neither agree nor disagree	Disagree	Can't choose/not answered
Many more streets in towns and cities should be reserved for pedestrians only	69	17	10	3
Banning company cars except where they are essential for employees in their work	53	19	25	5
The government should spend money on campaigns to persuade people to cut back on driving	39	28	24	8
The government should build more motorways to reduce traffic congestion	37	24	35	5
Drivers charged tolls on all motorways	24	21	51	5
Motorists charged for each mile they drive in city centres in working hours	18	21	57	4

Establishing priorities

The priorities in addressing the problems of the current transport system could therefore be described as firstly, tackling unnecessary car journeys, secondly providing safe, affordable and practical alternatives to the car — public transport, walking, cycling and thirdly, the introduction of disincentives to car use and incentives for other health promoting modes.

Although a range of measures to achieve the above have been discussed, clear evidence of efficacy in reducing the adverse impact of transport policy on health is lacking in many areas. Reviews of the clinical effectiveness of accident reduction strategies have identified a dearth of well designed trials to reduce road traffic accidents in young people, making it difficult to establish that specific measures would have the desired effect.[75,188] However, there is an important distinction between the potential effectiveness of an intervention, and the effectiveness demonstrated in a study of its particular humps used, or to transport patterns in the area, rather than proving road humps to be ineffective *per se*.

The lack of evidence makes it difficult to establish the key determinants for the use of certain modes of transport. It could be suggested that the population became less fit as a result of barriers to walking and cycling. Alternatively it could be that people are less inclined to use these transport modes because they have become less fit. However, conclusions can and should be drawn from the available evidence because for a number of the associations outlined in this report there are elements of both cause and effect. For example, less people cycle because of perceived danger with the result that motorists become less aware of cyclists and there are real increases in risks per cycle journey. There is also evidence from the UK and abroad that packages of measures including traffic calming, improve safety and increase levels of health promoting forms of transport.[50] It is reasonable to infer implications of policy changes from descriptive epidemiology describing variations over time, between locations within the UK, and by international comparisons. The available evidence is suggestive of a number of actions that can be taken in conjunction with ongoing research to assess efficacy and further improve knowledge.

Policy priorities

The examination of the health issues related to transport enable a number of policies to be proposed to reduce risk and promote health:

- support an integrated public transport system, with improved access to such modes and subsidies for family travel that discourage car use, for example, family tickets for public transport.

- promote further research into effective means of reducing the adverse health impact of road transport and ensure that road building and planning are assessed for their possible impacts on health.[189]

- reduce the number of people driving (perhaps target company car use over private motor use) through fiscal and traffic actual danger to pedestrians and cyclists. There is a growing volume of literature setting out traffic reduction strategies.[4,190,191]

- contain trip lengths so that walking and cycling are practical choices. This requires consistent implementation of Planning Policy Guidance Note 13, so as to reduce the need to travel,[14] (see page 12).

- change the street environment to deter inappropriate speeds by major investment in area wide traffic calming schemes. This requires substantially increasing expenditure on such measures, which have proved to be far more cost effective than measures to increase road capacity.

- promote positive images for walking and cycling as culturally acceptable modes of travel, as well as being environmentally benign and health promoting.

- promote strong intersectoral collaborative efforts across central government, and between health authorities, trusts, and other health sector staff including doctors, and with local government. Some 'Healthy Cities' and 'Health For All' initiatives, such as in Glasgow and Sheffield, have acknowledged the need for close intersectoral working on transport and health and are taking action; however, they remain exceptions.[192] The call to act 'for the public health' could provide the unifying theme for many interest groups.[193]

- provide easily accessible nationwide public transport information for bus as well as rail systems to publicise public transport availability and encourage greater use. A free-phone telephone system and the online opportunities of multi-media systems such as the Internet, would go some way towards tackling information deprivation. Visible and accurate timetables at stations, bus and tram stops are also needed, including the expansion of 'real time' information such as on the London Underground System, where information about the next service is given to the nearest minute.

6 Towards road transport and health

Increasing motor traffic is a most pressing problem in transport policy today. Strategies to reduce the harmful effects of motor cars such as emission controls are to be welcomed but will be outweighed by projected increases in motor traffic. There is therefore a need to consider reductions in motor traffic. Such reductions could lead to a broad range of health benefits. Physical and mental health and well being should be improved by reductions in air and noise pollution. Raising levels of physical activity in the population, and the health benefits this would confer, could be achieved by creating an environment in which walking and cycling are convenient, safe and easy options. The current transport system, however, does little to encourage and enable these modes. In fact the opposite is true and transport and planning policy has led more people to become dependent on the car, making the environment more hostile for others, including those in motor vehicles. This situation is neither cost-effective nor environmentally sustainable.

Developing an integrated transport system

Transport is a means to an end which is movement and access, but this should be at minimum cost to human health, the environment and the economy. Lower driving speeds, and land use planning to concentrate facilities at locations easily accessible by alternatives to the car, could bring overall benefits by enabling needs to be met more locally. Incorporating walking, cycling, and even driving to a certain extent, into a journey involving a mode of public transport into busy town/city centres. Major changes in policies and in funding towards low cost yet highly cost-effective traffic management schemes to encourage walking and cycling are also needed. By reducing reliance on motor transport an integrated and sustainable transport system could be developed that improves public health and —

- *reduces inequalities in health* by reducing inequities of access and improving local social support networks;

- *adds health to years of life* by reducing disease and disability resulting from both the directly quantifiable and the more cumulative impacts of transport on health;

- *add years to life* by reducing danger at source, pollution from motor traffic, and providing supportive environments which encourage physically active lifestyles, in turn promoting mental wellbeing;

— and by doing so, makes a key contribution to *The Health of the Nation* targets.[1]

Responsibility for developing and implementing healthy transport policy lies with many organisations, in a wide range of sectors. Government, both national and local, obviously has a key role and there is a need for a co-ordinated approach across Government and local authority departments. Indeed, the Government have recently announced their plans for a fundamental review of transport policy due to be published in a White Paper in Spring 1998. The European Commission has also launched an ambitious programme to promote road safety within the European Union. The Commission has asked Member States and all decision makers to take a systematic look at the cost of road accidents when deciding whether or not to invest in or take regulatory measures in favour of road safety. Some of the issues addressed include developing computer tools to manage traffic better and reducing the risk of accidents due to the consumption of alcohol, drugs or medicines.

The individual also has an important role in the choices they make regarding transport. Doctors and other health professionals are well placed to promote healthy transport policy individually with patients and collectively as part of a broader aim of promoting healthy public policy. Evidence suggests that health promotion

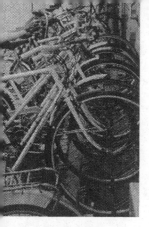

In the Netherlands, safe and appropriate facilities for walking and cycling, integrated with public transport are provided.

daily living;[194] and also add their voices to those calling for safer cycling and walking environments, not only in terms of safety from other vehicles, but also from being at risk of violence in isolated or poorly lit areas.[195] As the National Health Service is the largest employer in Great Britain it is important to lead by example and begin to change transport practices within the health sector. In 1996, the Department of Transport noted that the health sector was responsible for up to 5% of all trips, with two-thirds being made by people other than patients.[196] At a local level traffic reduction strategies are beginning to be developed by Health Authorities and Trusts, largely as a result of problems with car parking space and local authority planning refusal for increases.[197] A 'Healthy Transport Network' has been established by Transport 2000 which produces a regular newsletter for Trusts and Health Authorities.[198] There are now more than 80 members, all with an interest in reducing car trips to health facilities. A newsletter specifically focusing on the promotion of cycling in the health sector has also been produced by the 'Bike for Your Life' project.[199] It is not just the NHS, however, that is responsible, all organisations have a role to play by introducing a healthy transport plan or 'Green Commuter Plan' to encourage staff to use more health promoting forms of transport.[200]

This report serves to highlight the many ways in which transport policy affects health and outlines some possible solutions. It will be the job of transport planners to develop new approaches that take into account such factors in order that the UK may move towards an equitable, sustainable and health promoting transport system.

Targets for changes in reliance on different transport modes

Transport targets to promote health need to do more than just seek increases in travel by walking, public transport, and cycling, such as the doubling of cycling trips by 2002.[56] The Department of the Environment, Transport and the Regions has yet to be convinced of a net benefit from national road traffic targets to reduce car use unless there is widespread consensus among local authorities.[201] This may, however, be forthcoming, given that local authorities

Road Traffic Reduction Bill was presented to Parliament in November 1996, and has, after some amendment, become an Act of Parliament. This reveals the growing concern about traffic volumes and congestion. Unfortunately, however, even though the Act requires local and regional traffic targets to be set, it does not require the national targets as stated in the original Bill. Until motor traffic growth is halted and reversed, targets for increasing levels of walking and cycling are likely to be hindered by street environments dominated by motorized traffic. Targets must be set for absolute and relative reductions in the number of trips and kilometres travelled by motor vehicles and heavy goods vehicles. Motor traffic reduction is a crucial issue to releasing the potential demand for walking and cycling (including connections to public transport).

Recommendations

Department of the Environment, Transport and the Regions (DETR):

- ensure that the structure of the newly merged Department reflects the fundamentally different approach which a sustainable and health promoting transport policy requires so that environmental concerns take the lead;

- establish health derived national motor traffic reduction targets;

- establish a Traffic Reduction Unit, headed by a senior civil servant, reporting directly to the Secretary of State, to co-ordinate action to achieve traffic reduction targets;

- establish stringent limits on emissions for diesel vehicles and encourage more research on catalysts for diesel vehicles to reduce particulate matter and nitrogen oxides;

- establish health derived traffic noise pollution reduction targets as part of a revised national Environmental Health Action Plan, by setting targets on engine and exhaust noise via the vehicle test (MoT) and setting targets on tyre noise reduction programmes;

transport connections and thus increasing the public transport catchment (40% of rail trips in the Netherlands start or finish as a bicycle trip). This should include free provision for bicycles on buses, as commonly found elsewhere in Europe and parts of the United States (eg. Seattle), and on trains, through franchise agreements;

- consider mechanisms (eg. financial) to restrict the use of heavy goods vehicles;

- encourage a modal shift to rail freight by reassessing the rail freight grants eligibility conditions and application procedures and widely promote the availability of the grants;

- recommend that transport operators provide bicycle parks at all major public transport interchanges;

- establish a Children's unit responsible for encouraging and guiding local authorities in the development of 'Safe Routes to Schools' initiatives, focusing on keeping children safe from traffic and 'stranger danger' (see page 45). This must involve close liaison with staff working on traffic calming programmes, those planning new housing estates, the Departments of Health and Education and school representative bodies, including those representing staff and police;

- establish through the National Walking Strategy Steering Group health derived targets for increases in walking, according to age group;

- establish traffic danger reduction targets, using as indicators of progress the percentage of children travelling to school by foot and by bike set against casualty rates (especially for 10-14 year olds);

- meet the objective of the National Cycling Strategy to double the number of school children cycling to school whilst still maintaining an awareness of safe cycle routes;

- develop more rigorous enforcement of speed limits and increase the use of speed cameras etc;

- provide increased funding for local authority 20 mph schemes and to approve a minimum of 500 additional 20mph zones by the year 2002, and to set targets for further increases thereafter;

access to public transport, and to give further consideration to the needs of disabled people and the elderly in terms of the road environment — tactile paving, for example;

- improve driver training to include hazard perception and awareness of cycling, particularly in younger drivers. This could involve, for example, the introduction of a practical cycling section in the Driving Test;

- investigate the cost effectiveness for uniform in-car speed limiters in terms of environmental and health benefits;

- include community and voluntary transport and financing issues in Transport Policies and Programmes Package Bids and review funding criteria for the Rural Transport Development Fund with a two-tier approach to provide higher levels of assistance to areas with low population densities;

- work with the Department of Trade and Industry to develop more energy efficient vehicles with top speeds which reflect UK speed limits;

- encourage and promote the use of electric vehicles (eg. trams) within the urban land space;

- approach insurance companies with regard to their policies on multiple-users and petrol-cost sharing which at present invalidates policy;

- promote mileage related car insurance;

- target commercial organisations and encourage them to publish and disseminate their transport policies;

- reduce the permitted blood alcohol concentration (BAC) for driving to 50mg/100ml;

- press for legislation at European Union level in order to harmonise the permitted BACs to no more than 50mg/100ml;

- introduce highly visible and well publicised roadside random breath testing;

- support consistently the aims of Planning Policy Guidance Note 13 and continue to monitor its effectiveness in reducing the need for motorized transport through planning and location of facilities (see page 12).

- consider the feasibility of the abolition of the Vehicle Excise Duty and the transfer of costs on to fuel duty and other taxes on cars, motoring and related activities so as to discourage unnecessary car and heavy goods vehicle use. However, the adverse effects of such measures for the disabled or those in rural areas must be considered;
- remove tax concessions on company cars;
- introduce concessions for health promoting forms of transport such as cycles and equipment, discounted public transport season tickets as part of employers 'green commuter' plans.

Department of Education:

- ensure road safety is considered as part of the national curriculum;
- monitor implementation and efficacy of road safety education and health education with regards to transport in schools;
- encourage 'Walk to School' campaigns.

Department of Health:

- work with the Departments of the Environment, Transport, and the Regions, and Education in promoting the personal health benefits of walking and cycling, children and adolescents should be encouraged to develop physically active lifestyles from early childhood. This work should include developing guidelines for involving health promotion staff and the encouragement of 'Safe Routes to Schools' initiatives;
- contribute to the development of a health audit to assess the health impact of new transport infrastructure which should be considered alongside traditional transport cost benefit analysis;
- adopt the 'precautionary principle' where evidence of beneficial or adverse effects of road transport on health is incomplete, giving the benefit of the doubt to protecting health and the environment;
- continue to research and monitor the medical effects of air pollution and other health effects of transport policies.

- establish road user hierarchies which place pedestrians, people with mobility restrictions, and cyclists at the top and car borne commuters as the bottom, as adopted in cities such as York and Oxford;
- give consideration to city centre car bans;
- develop safe and appropriate facilities for walking and cycling, integrated with public transport;
- address the need for a co-ordinated approach to road safety education for young people utilizing the Transport Research Laboratory Code of Good Practice in Road Safety in Schools[202] and Local Authorities Association Roads Safety Code of Good Practice.

NHS Executive:

- set a national target to reduce the contribution of the health sector to motorized trips;
- when issuing guidance on accessibility when health facilities relocate, emphasise that health facilities should be planned to be accessible to staff, patients and visitors by public transport, foot and bicycle whilst strongly discouraging car use, eg. changing bus routes to health service facilities;
- develop and issue guidelines on minimum cycle parking standards and maximum car parking standards at health facilities.

Health Authorities/Trusts:

- develop partnerships with local authorities and public transport operators to improve public transport access to health service facilities;
- set targets, draw up and promote 'healthy transport plans' to encourage a shift from cars to other transport modes amongst staff and visitors, eg. public transport subsidies and targeting schemes such as 'Ring and Ride'.

- promote physically active lifestyles, such as walking and cycling;

- monitor and report on the effects of transport policy on health, in particular through the Annual Reports of Directors of Public Health;

- consider transport and access in locating health facilities;

- as individuals with a key role in preventing ill health, be exemplary in terms of modes of transport used.

Organisations (including the BMA):

- introduce a 'Green Commuter Plan' or healthy transport plan to encourage staff to use more health promoting forms of transport;[199,200,201,203]

- offer staff a travel pass giving a reduction on bus routes;

- provide easily accessible local public transport information (timetables etc);

- organise 'Park and Ride' schemes;

- organise shuttle bus services from local public transport stations;

- organise and promote a car pool scheme and offer preferential parking for those sharing;

- increase car park charges for those not sharing and invest the extra money into improved public transport facilities;

- offer staff interest free loans to purchase a bicycle;

- provide adequate cycle parking facilities, lockers and also shower facilities;

- allow staff who cycle in the course of work to claim a larger amount per mile than if they were to undertake the journey by car;

- purchase several bicycles for staff to rent for a small fee per week or allow members of staff to sign up for a year at no charge if they surrender parking permits;

- arrange for any bicycle repairs to be done on site during working hours and where not possible — offer a replacement bicycle until repairs can be completed.

7 References

1 Department of Health. *The Health of the Nation: A strategy for health in England*. London: HMSO, 1992

2 Central Statistical Office. *Social Trends*. London: HMSO, 1997

3 Central Statistical Office. *Social Trends*. London: HMSO, 1996

4 Royal Commission on Environmental Pollution. *18th Report: Transport and the environment*. London: HMSO, 1994

5 The Observer. *Blueprint for a National Travel Plan to take Britain's Transport System into the 21st Century*. London: The Observer, (Undated)

6 Royal Automobile Club. *Summary Report: Car dependence*. London: RAC, 1995

7 Department of Transport. *Journey Times Survey*. London: HMSO, 1997

8 Department of Transport. *National Travel Survey: 1992/94*. London: HMSO, 1995

9 Department of Transport. *National Travel Survey: 1989/91*. London: HMSO, 1993

10 Department of the Environment. *Sustainable Development: The UK strategy*. London: HMSO, 1994

11 Department of Transport. *Transport Statistics Great Britain*. London: HMSO, 1995

12 Morris B, Snelson A, Watters P, Lawson, S. The journey to work: Reports and Stated Preference of 2520 Automobile Association employees and their response to a car-sharing initiative. *Traffic Engineering and Control* 1992;33(11):619-624

13 Department of the Environment, Scottish Office. *The United Kingdom National Air Quality Strategy. Consultation draft*. London: DOE, 1996

14 Department of the Environment, Department of Transport. *Planning Policy Guidance Note 13: Transport*. London: HMSO, 1994

15 Countryside Commission. *Trends in Transport and the Countryside*. Cheltenham: Countryside Commission, 1992

16 Department of the Environment. *Digest of Environmental Protection and Water Statistics*. London: HMSO, 1994

18 University of Westminster. *Public Attitudes to Transport Policy and the Environment: An in-depth exploratory study. Summary Report to the Department of Transport.* London: Transport Studies Group, University of Westminster, 1996

19 Jowell R et al (eds). *British Social Attitudes.* Aldershot: Dartmouth Publishing, 1996

20 Activity and Health Research. *Allied Dunbar National Fitness Survey.* London: Health Education Authority and Sports Council, 1992

21 National Forum for Coronary Heart Disease Prevention. *Physical Activity: An agenda for action.* London: NFCHDP, 1995

22 Morris JN. Exercise in the prevention of coronary heart disease: today's best buy in public health. *Medicine and Science in Sports and Exercise* 1994;26:807-814

23 Prentice AM, Jebb SA. Obesity in Britain: gluttony or sloth? *British Medical Journal* 1995;311:437-9

24 Department of Health. *Strategy Statement on Physical Activity.* London: DOH, 1996

25 Pedestrians' Policy Group. *Walking Forward.* London: Transport 2000 Trust, Undated

26 World Health Organisation, International Federation of Sports Medicine. Exercise for Health: WHO/IFSM Committee on physical activity for health. *Bulletin of the World Health Organisation* 1995;73:135-136

27 United States Department of Health and Human Services. *Physical Activity and Health: A report of the Surgeon General.* Atlanta,GA: US Department of Health and Human Services, 1997

28 Morris J, Clayton D, Everitt M, Semmence A, Burgess E. Exercise in Leisure Time: Coronary attack and death rates. *British Heart Journal* 1990;63:325-334

29 Paffenbarger R, Hyde R, Wing A, Hsieh C. Physical Activity, All-Cause Mortality, and Longevity of College Alumni. *New England Journal of Medicine* 1986;314:605-613

30 Oja P, Manttari A, Heinonen A, Kukkonen-Harjula K, Laukkanen R, Pasanen M, Vuori I. Physiological Effects of Walking and Cycling to Work. *Scandinavian Journal of Medicine, Science in Sports* 1991;1:151-157

31 Vuori I, Oja P, Paronen O. Physically Active Commuting to Work — Testing its potential for exercise promotion. *Medicine and Science in Sports and Exercise* 1994;26:844-850

32 Young A, Dinan S. ABC of sports medicine. Fitness for older people. *British Medical Journal* 1994;309:331-334

33 Brown M, Holloszy J. Effects of walking, jogging and cycling on strength, flexibility, speed and balance in 60 to 72 year olds. *Ageing Clinical and Experimental Research* 1993;5:427-434

34 Greendale G, Barrett-Connor E, Edelstein S, Haile R. Lifetime leisure exercise and osteoporosis: The Rancho Bernardo study. *American Journal of Epidemiology* 1995;141:951-959

37   Tuxworth B. *The health benefits of walking. Part 1 of a submission 'The Value of Walking', to the Consultation Paper 'More People More Active More Often'*. London: Transport and Health Study Group, 1995

38   Norris R, Carroll D, Cochrane R. The Effects of Physical Activity and Exercise Training on Psychological Stress and Wellbeing in an Adolescent Population. *Journal of Psychosomatic Research* 1992;36:55-65

39   Steptoe A, Butler N. Sports Participation and Emotional Wellbeing in Adolescents. *Lancet* 1996;347:1789-1792

40   Cramer S, Nieman D, Lee J. The Effects of Moderate Exercise Training on Psychological Wellbeing and Mood State in Women. *Journal of Psychosomatic Research* 1991;35:437-449

41   Byrne A, Byrne D. The Effect of Exercise on Depression, Anxiety and Other Mood States: A review. *Journal of Psychosomatic Research* 1993;37:565-574

42   Cyclists' Touring Club. *Bikes not Fumes*. Godalming:CTC, 1991

43   British Medical Association. *Cycling: Towards Health & Safety*. Oxford: Oxford University Press, 1992

44   Department of Transport. *Cycling in Great Britain - Transport Statistics Report*. London: HMSO, 1996

45   Cyclists' Touring Club, Bicycle Association, Department of Transport, Institution of Highways and Transportation. *Cycle-friendly Infrastructure - Guidelines for Planning and Design*, Godalming:CTC, 1996

46   Hillman M. Cycling and the Promotion of Health. *Policy Studies* 1993;14:49-58

47   Tuxworth W, Neville AM, White C, Jenkins C. Health, fitness, physical activity and morbidity of middle aged male factory workers. *British Journal of Industrial Medicine* 1986;43:733-753

48   Hendriksen I. *The Effect of Commuter Cycling on Physical Performance and on Coronary Heart Disease Risk Factors*. Amsterdam: Free University, 1997

49   Hillman, M. Health promotion and non-motorized transport. In Fletcher T, McMichael AJ (eds). *Health at the Crossroads — Transport policy and urban health*. Sussex: J Wiley and Sons, 1997

50   Cyclists' Touring Club. *More Bikes - Policy into best practice*. Godalming: CTC, 1995

51   Mynors P, Savell A. *Cycling on the Continent*. London: Travers Morgan Transport, 1992

52   Transport Committee. *Transport Committee Third Report: Risk reduction for vulnerable road users*. London: HMSO, 1996

53   Local Transport Today. 25 Nov 1993:13

54   Transport Research Laboratory. *Review of Traffic Calming Schemes in 20 mph Zones, Report 215*. Crowthorne: Transport Research Laboratory, 1996

56 Department of Transport. *The National Cycling Strategy.* London: HMSO, 1996

57 Department of Transport. *Developing a Strategy for Walking.* London: DOT, 1996

58 Davis A. Livable streets and perceived accident risk: quality of life issues for residents and vulnerable road users. *Traffic Engineering and Control* 1992;33:374-387

59 Department of Transport. *Road Accidents Great Britain 1995.* London: HMSO, 1996

60 Department of Transport. *Road Casualties Great Britain: Final Figures 1996.* London: HMSO, 1997

61 Hillman M, Adams J, Whitelegg J. *One False Move: A study of children's independent mobility.* London: Policy Studies Institute, 1991

62 Roberts I. Why have child pedestrian death rates fallen? *British Medical Journal* 1993;306:1737-1739

63 Road Danger Reduction Forum. *Is It Safe? A guide to road danger reduction.* Leeds:RDRF,Undated

64 DiGuiseppi C, Roberts I, Leah L. Influence of changing travel patterns on child death rates from injury: Trend analysis. *British Medical Journal* 1997;314:710-3.

65 Ward H, Care J, Morrison A et al. *Pedestrian Activity and Accident Risk.* Basingstoke: AA Foundation for Road Safety Research, 1994

66 West-Oram F. Measuring danger on the road. *Traffic Engineering and Control* 1989;30(10):529-532

67 Monheim H. Spielrume des Kommenunalen Strassenbaus. *Stressen und Tiefbau.* Heft 1, 2 and 3, Isenhagen, Germany, 1984

68 Department of Transport. *Road Safety Casualty Reduction - Targeting the future.* London: DOT, 1996

69 Cyclists' Touring Club, Pedestrians Association. *Joint Statement on Providing for Walking and Cycling as Transport and Travel.* Godalming: CTC, 1995

70 Sabey B. *Road Safety into the '80's Symposium: Recent developments and research in road safety remedial measures.* Manchester: University of Salford, 1983

71 Carson O, Tight M, Southwell M, Plows B. *Urban accidents: Why do they happen?* Basingstoke: Automobile Association Foundation for Road Safety Research, 1989

72 Finch D, Kompfner P, Lockwood C, Maycock G. *Speed, Speed Limits and Accidents. Project Report 58.* Crowthorne: Transport Research Laboratory, 1994

73 Department of Transport. *Vehicle Speeds in Great Britain 1995 - Statistics Bulletin (96)31.* London: HMSO, 1996

74 Department of the Environment, Transport and the Regions. *Vehicle speeds in Great Britain: 1996,* London: HMSO, 1997

75 Coleman P et al. *The Effectiveness of Interventions to Prevent Accidental Injury to Young Persons Aged 15-24 Years: A review of the evidence.* Sheffield: Sheffield Centre for Health and Related Research, 1996

Velocity Conference Proceedings. Nottingham: Nottinghamshire County Council, 1994

77   Plowden S, Hillman M. *Speed Control and Transport Policy.* London: Policy Studies Institute, 1996

78   Department of Transport. *Transport Statistics Great Britain 1995.* London: HMSO, 1996

79   British Medical Association. *Driving Impairment through Alcohol and other Drugs.* London: BMA, 1996

80   Poloniecki JD, Atkinson RW, Ponce de Leon A, Anderson HR. Daily time series for cardiovascular hospital admissions and previous day's air pollution in London, UK. *Occupational and Environmental Medicine* 1997;54:535-540

81   Wjst M, Reitmeir P, Dold S, Wulff A, Nicolai T, von Loeffelholz-Colberg E, von Matius E. Road traffic and adverse effects on respiratory health in children. *British Medical Journal* 1993;307:596-600

82   Raaschou-Nielsen O, Nielsen M, Gehl J. Traffic-Related Air Pollution: Exposure to health effects in Copenhagen street cleaners and cemetery workers. *Archives of Environmental Health* 1995;50:207-220

83   Abbey D, Hwang B, Buchette R., Vancuren T, Mills P. Estimated Long-Term Ambient Concentrations of PM_{10} and Development of Respiratory Symptoms in a Nonsmoking Population. *Archives of Environmental Health* 1995;50:139-152

84   Quality of Urban Air Review Group. *Airborne Particulate Matter in the UK.* Birmingham: University of Birmingham Institute of Public and Environmental Health, 1996

85   Savitz D, Feingold L. Association of Childhood Cancer with Residential Traffic Density. *Scandinavian Journal of Work, Environment and Health* 1989;15:360-363

86   Guerra G, Iemma D, Lerda C, Martines C. Benziene Emissions from Motor Vehicle Traffic in the Urban Area of Milan: Hypothesis of health impact assessment. *Atmospheric Environment* 1995;29:3559-3569

87   World Health Organisation. *Air Quality Guidelines for Europe - Series 23.* Copenhagen: Regional Office for Europe, 1987

88   Mathew D, Rowell A. *The Environmental Impact of the Car.* London: Greenpeace International, 1991

89   International Agency for Research on Cancer. *Diesel and Gasoline Engine Exhaust and Some Nitroarenes - Monograph on the Evaluation of Carcinogenic Risk in Humans, Vol. 46.* Lyon: IARC, 1989

90   Forastiere F et al. Mortality Among Urban Policemen in Rome. *American Journal of Industrial Medicine* 1994;26:785-798

91   Van Den Eeden S, Friedman G. Exposure to Engine Exhaust and Risk of Subsequent Cancer. *Journal of Occupational Medicine* 1993;35:307-311

92   International Panel on Climate Change. *Climate Change 1995.* Cambridge: Cambridge University Press, 1996

94 Krommendijk E. *Bicycle and Environment in the City: A quantification of some environmental effects of a bicycle orientated traffic policy in Groningen.* Groningen: Prof HC van Hall Institute, 1988

95 Jefferiss P, Rowell A, Fergusson M. *The Exposure of Car Drivers and Passengers to Vehicle Emissions; Comparative pollutant levels inside and outside vehicles. A Report For Greenpeace UK by Earth Resources Research.* London: Greenpeace, 1992

96 Wijen J, Verhoeff A, Jans H, Bruggen M. The Exposure of Cyclists, Car Drivers and Pedestrians to Traffic-Related Air Pollutants. *International Archives of Occupational and Environmental Health* 1995;67:187-193

97 Department of the Environment, Department of Health, Department of Transport. *Health Effects of Particles. The Government's preliminary response to the reports of the Committee on the Medical Effects of Air Pollutants and the Expert Panel on Air Quality Standards.*. London: DOE, 1995

98 Bates D. Air Pollution: Time for More Clean Air Legislation. *British Medical Journal* 1996;312:649-650

99 Van Den Hout KD, Rijkeboer RC. *Diesel Exhaust and Air Pollution.* Delft: Research Institute for Road Vehicles, 1986

100 'ERGA Air Pollution' Ad hoc Group. *Present and Future Air Quality in the United Kingdom and the Relative Responsibility of Motor Vehicles. Report. No 11/602/83-EN-FINAL, Annex 3, Document 34.* Brussels: ERGA Air Pollution, 1983

101 Department of Health. *Non-Biological Particles and Health.* London: HMSO, 1995

102 Utell M, Samet J. Particulate Air Pollution and Health: New evidence on an old problem. *American Review of Respiratory Disease* 1993;147:1334-1335

103 Seaton A, MacNee W, Donaldson K, Godden D. Particulate Air Pollution and Acute Health Effects. *Lancet* 1995;345:176-178

104 Walters S. What are the respiratory health effects of vehicle pollution? In: Read C (ed) *How vehicle pollution affects our health.* London: Ashden Trust, 1994

105 Dockery DW, Pope CA, Xu X et al. An Association between Air pollution and Mortality in 6 US Cities. *New England Journal of Medicine* 1993;329:1753-1759

106 Parliamentary Office of Science and Technology. *Breathing in our cities.* London:POST, 1994

107 Edwards J, Walters S, Griffiths, R. Hospital Admissions for Asthma in Preschool Children: Relationship to Major Roads in Birmingham, United Kingdom. *Archives of Environmental Health* 1994;49:223-227

108 Weiland S, Mundt K, Ruckmann S, Keil U. Self-Reported Wheezing and Allergic Rhinitis in Children and Traffic Density on Street of Residence. *Annals of Epidemiology* 1994;4:243-247

109 Oosterlee A, Drijver M, Lebret E, Brunekreef B. Chronic Respiratory Symptoms in Children and Adults Living along Streets with High Traffic Density. *Occupational and Environmental Medicine* 1996;53:241-247

110 Department of Health. *Asthma and Outdoor Air Pollution.* London: HMSO, 1995

Environment 1995;169:71-74

112 Whitelegg J, Gatrell A, Newmann P. *Traffic and Health*. Lancaster: University of Lancaster Environmental Epidemiology Research Unit, 1993

113 Department of the Environment, Department of Health. *Consultative Document: The Environment and Health*. London:DOE, 1996

114 World Health Organisation. *Concern for Europe's Tomorrow: Health and the environment in the WHO European region*. Stuttgart: European Centre for Environment and Health, 1995

115 Sargent J, Fothergill L. *The Noise Climate Around Our Homes. Information Paper IP21/93*. Watford: Building Research Establishment, 1993

116 Ohrstrom E, Rylander R. Sleep Disturbance by Road Traffic Noise - A laboratory study on number of noise events. *Journal of Sound and Vibration* 1990;143:93-101

117 Eberhardt J. The Influence of Road Traffic Noise on Sleep. *Journal of Sound and Vibration* 1988;127:449-455

118 Carter N. Transportation Noise, Sleep, and Possible After-Effects. *Environment International* 1996;22:105-116

119 Ohrstrom E. Psycho-Social Effects of Traffic Noise Exposure. *Journal of Sound and Vibration* 1991;151:513-517

120 Health and Safety Executive. *Noise at Work Regulations 1989*. London: HMSO, 1990

121 Institute of Environmental Health Officers. *Transportation: The route to health report*. London: IEHO, 1993

122 Lercher P, Kofler W. Behavioural and Health Responses Associated with Road Traffic Noise Exposure along Alpine Through-Traffic Routes. *Science of the Total Environment* 1996;189/190:85-89

123 Department of the Environment. *The United Kingdom National Environmental Health Action Plan*. London: HMSO, 1996

124 Franks P, Campbell T, Shields C. Social Relationships and Health: The relative roles of family functioning and social support. *Social Science and Medicine* 1992;34:779-788

125 Berkman L, Syme L. Social Networks, Host Resistance, and Mortality: A nine-year follow-up study of Alameda County residents. *American Journal of Epidemiology* 1979;109:186-204

126 Casell J. The Contribution of the Social Environment to Host Resistance. *American Journal of Epidemiology* 1976;104:107-123

127 Welin L, Tibblin G, Svrdsudd K, Tibblin B, Ander-Peciva S, Larsson B, Wilhelmsen L. Prospective Study of Social Influences on Mortality. The study of men born in 1913 and 1923. *Lancet* 1985;1(8434):915-918

128 Fox J. Social network interaction: new jargon in health inequalities. *British Medical Journal* 1988;297:373-374

130 Greenwood DC, Muir KR, Packham CJ, Madeley RJ. Coronary heart disease: a review of the role of psychosocial stress and social support. *Journal of Public Health Medicine* 1996;18:221-31

131 Clarke JM et al. *The Appraisal of Community Severance - Transport Road Research Laboratory Contractor Report 135.* Crowthorne: Transport Road Research Laboratory, 1991

132 Morrissey C, Hedges B. *Adaptation to Increases in Traffic Exposure - Transport Road Research Laboratory Contractor Report 245.* Crowthorne: Transport Road Research Laboratory, 1991

133 Appleyard D, Lintell M. The Environmental Quality of City Streets: The residents' viewpoint. *American Institute of Planners Journal* 1972;38:84-101

134 Klæboe R. *Measuring the Environmental Impact of Road Traffic in Town Areas. Paper to PTRC Summer Annual Meeting, Seminar B, pp 81-88* London: PTRC, 1992

135 Hine J, Russell J. The Impact of Traffic on Pedestrian Behaviour: Assessing the traffic barrier on radial routes. *Traffic Engineering and Control* 1996;32(2):81-85

136 Danish Road Directorate. *Consequence Evaluation of Environmentally Adapted Through Road in Vinderu - Report 52.* Herlev:Road Data Laboratory,1987

137 Transport Research Laboratory. *Survey of Public Acceptability of a Traffic Management Scheme in Sheffield. RSL Report for Transport Research Laboratory.* Crowthorne: Transport Research Laboratory, 1992

138 Taylor D. *Public Attitudes and Consultation in Traffic Calming Schemes, Doctoral Thesis.* Leeds: Institute of Transport Studies, University of Leeds, 1995

139 London Strategic Policy Unit. *Women's Safe Transport in London.* London: London Strategic Policy Unit, 1988

140 Valentine G. The Geography of Women's Fear. *Area* 1989;21:385-390

141 Maddison D, Pearce D, Johansson O, Calthorp E, Litman T, Verhoef E. *The True Costs of Road Transport, Blueprint 5.* London: Centre for Social and Economic Research on the Global Environment, 1996

142 Sustrans. *Safety on the Streets for Children. Information Sheet FF10.* Bristol: Sustrans, 1996

143 Nicholl J, Freeman M, Williams B. Effects of Subsidising Bus Travel on the Occurrence of Road Traffic Casualties. *Journal of Epidemiology and Community Health* 1987;41:50-54

144 Hamilton K, Jenkins L, Gregory A. *Women and Transport: Bus de-regulation in West Yorkshire.* Bradford: University of Bradford, 1991

145 Sheffield City Council. *The Bus Booklet.* Sheffield:SCC,1986

146 Department of Transport. *Bus and Coach Statistics Great Britain 1993-1994.* London: HMSO, 1994

147 Rural Development Commission. *Community and Voluntary Transport in Rural England.* Salisbury: RDC, 1996

149 Banister D. *Transport mobility and deprivation in inner urban areas.* Farnborough: Gower, 1980

150 National Forum for Coronary Heart Disease Prevention. *Food for Children.* London: NFCHDP, 1993

151 Piachaud D, Webb J. *The Price of Food.*, London: London School of Economics, 1996

152 Leather S. Less Money, Less Choice: Poverty and diet in the UK today. In: *Your Food: Whose choice?* London: National Consumer Council, 1992

153 Morton S, Hannah J. 'Within Minutes of the M62' - Major Retail Development Proposals for Great Manchester. *Radical Community Medicine* 1989;38:28-33

154 Townsend P, Davidson N (eds). *Inequalities in Health: The Black Report.* London: Penguin, 1988

155 British Medical Association. *Inequalities in Health.* London: BMA, 1995

156 Benzeval M, Judge K, Whitehead M (eds) *Tackling Inequalities in Health: An agenda for action.* London: Kings Fund, 1995

157 General Household Survey. *Living in Britain: Results from the General Household Survey 1994 OPCS.* London: HMSO, 1996

158 Grieco M. *Low Income Families and Inter-Household Interdependency: The implications for transport policy and planning - Paper to Transport and Urban deprivation workshop.* Liverpool: University of Liverpool, 1989

159 Bindman A et al. Preventable Hospitalisations and Access to Health Care. *Journal of the American Medical Association* 1995;274:305-311

160 Greater London Association of Disabled People. *All Change 2000: The Report.* London: Greater London Association of Disabled People, 1996

161 Roberts I, Power C. Does the decline in child injury mortality vary by social class? *British Medical Journal* 1996;313:784-786

162 Roberts I, Norton R, Taua B. Child pedestrian injury rates: the importance of 'exposure to risk' relating to socioeconomic and ethnic differences in Auckland, New Zealand. *Journal of Epidemiology and Community Health* 1996;50:162-165

163 Stevenson M, Jamrozik K, Spittle J. A Case-Control Study of Traffic Risk Factors and Child Pedestrian Injury. *International Journal of Epidemiology* 1995;24:957-964

164 Mueller B, Rivara F, Lii S, Weiss N. Environmental Factors and the Risk for Childhood Pedestrian-Motor Vehicle Collision Occurrence. *American Journal of Epidemiology* 1990;132:550-560

165 Bagley C. The Urban Environment and Child Pedestrian and Bicycle Injuries: Interaction of ecological and personality characteristics. *Journal of Community and Applied Social Psychology* 1992;2:281-289

166 Roberts I. Who's Prepared for Advocacy? Another inverse law. *Injury Prevention* 1995;1:152-154

168 British Association for Community Child Health. *Cars and Child Health - Briefing Paper*. London: BACCH, 1996

169 Davis A, Jones L. Environmental Constraints on Health: Listening to children's views. *The Health Education Journal* 1996;55:363-374

170 Davis A, Jones L. Children in the urban environment: an issue for the new public health agenda. *Health and Place* 1996;2:107-113

171 Jarvis S, Towner E, Walsh S. Accidents. In: Botting B (ed.) *The Health of Our Children*. London: HMSO, 1995

172 Gaster, S. Urban Children's Access to their Neighbourhood: Changes over three generations. *Environment and Behaviour* 1991;23:70-85

173 Cale L, Almond L. Physical activity levels of secondary school-aged children: A review. *Health Education Journal* 1992;51/4;192-197

174 Armstrong N, McManus N. Children's Fitness and Physical Activity - A challenge for Physical Education. *British Journal of Physical Education* 1994;25(1):20-26

175 Sleap M, Warburton P. Physical Activity Levels of 5-11 year-old children in England: Cumulative evidence from three direct observation studies. *International Journal of Sports Medicine* 1996;17:248-253

176 Chartered Society of Physiotherapy. *Physiotherapists concerned about unfit, fat, flabby young people*. Press Release: 26th June 1995

177 Kuhl D, Cooper C. Physical activity at 36 years: patterns and childhood predictors in a longitudinal study. *Journal of Epidemiology and Community Health* 1992;46:114-119

178 Raitakari O, Porkka K, Taimela S, Telma R., Rsnen L, Viikari J. Effects of persistent physical activity and inactivity on coronary risk factors in children and young adults. *American Journal of Epidemiology* 1994;140:195-205

179 Harsha D. The benefits of physical activity in childhood. *American Journal of the Medical Sciences* 1995;310:S109-113

180 Kegerreis S. Independent mobility and child mental and emotional development. In: Hillman M (ed). *Children, Transport and the Quality of Life*. London: Policy Studies Institute, 1993

181 Noschis J. Child development theory and planning for neighbourhood play. *Children's Environments* 1992;9:3-9

182 Health Education Authority. *Health promotion in childhood and young adolescence for the prevention of unintentional injuries*. HEA: London, 1996

183 Fowkes A, Oxley P, Heiser B. *Cross-sector benefits of accessible public transport*. Cranfield: University School of Management, 1994

184 Roper T, Mulley G. Caring for Older People: Public transport. *British Medical Journal* 1996;313:415-418

185 Gallon C, Fowkes A, Edwards M. *Accidents Involving Visually Impaired People using Public Transport or Walking*. Crowthorne: Transport Research Laboratory, 1995

187 Lowe M. Cycling into the future. In: Browne LR (ed). *State of the World 1990. A Worldwatch Institute report on progress towards a sustainable society.* New York: W W Norton, 1990

188 Nuffield Institute for Health. Preventing Unintentional Injuries in Children and Young Adolescents. *Effective Health Care* 1996;2:1-16

189 Joffe M, Sutcliffe J. Developing Policies for a Healthy Environment. *Health Promotion International.* 1997;12(2):169-173

190 Friends of the Earth. *Less Traffic Better Towns.* London: Friends of the Earth, 1992

191 Engwicht D. *Towards an Eco-City: Calming the traffic.* Sydney: Envirobook, 1992

192 Davis A. *Transport as Healthy Public Policy.* Liverpool: Health For All Network News, 1995

193 Jones L. *Transport and Health: The next move. Policy Statement on Transport.* London: Association for Public Health, 1994

194 Bike For Your Life. *Cycling as Physical Activity: A report of a questionnaire survey of health promotion and public health staff in England.* Nuneaton:Bike For Your Life, 1996

195 Health of Londoners Project. *Transport in London and the Implications for Health.* London: East London and The City Health Authority, 1996

196 Department of Transport. *Transport Secretary Urges Hospitals to Reduce Reliance on the Car. Press Notice 291.* London: DoT, 17 September 1996

197 Owen L, Davis A. Life Cycle: What are Trusts doing to encourage healthier transport practices? *The Health Service Journal* 1995; 24 August:26-27

198 Transport 2000 Trust. *Healthy Transport Newsletter.* London: Transport 2000, November 1996

199 Bike for Your Life. *Reaping the Benefits: A Cycling and Health Resource Pack.* Surrey: Cyclists' Touring Club, 1997

200 Transport 2000 Trust, London First. *Changing Journeys to Work: An employers' guide to green commuter plans.* London:Transport 2000, 1997

201 Department of Transport. *Transport: The way forward.* London: HMSO, 1996

202 Harland DG, Murray G, Tucker S. *Road Safety Education: Making safe connections. Paper presented at Safety '91.* Crowthorne: Transport Research Laboratory, 1991

203 London Cycling Campaign. *Cycling Charter for Employers.* Unpublished, 1991

8 Index

Scientific Publications

Title	Price
A Code of Practice for Implementation of the UK Hepatitis B Immunisation Guidelines for the Protection of Patients and Staff	£4.95
A Guide to Hepatitis C	£5.95
AIDS and You - Illustrated Guide	£2.25
Cycling: Towards Health and Safety	£5.99
Infection Control	£7.95
Multicultural Health Care: Current Practice and Future Policy	£6.95
Reporting Adverse Drug Reactions	£5.95
Sport and Exercise Medicine: Policy and Provision	£6.95
The BMA Guide to Living with Risk	£5.95
The BMA Guide to Rabies	£17.50
The Boxing Debate	£6.95
The Misuse of Drugs	£12.99
Water: A Vital Resource	£6.95

These publications can be obtained in person from the:

BMJ Bookshop, BMA House, Tavistock Square, London WC1H 9JP

or by post from the:

BMJ Bookshop, PO Box 295, London WC1H 9TE
Cheques should be made payable to the **BMJ Bookshop.**

or by telephone on: 0171 383 6185

Discounts are available to BMA members. Prices include p&p on UK orders only.